I0393872

Evidence Synthesis
Number 114

Behavioral Sexual Risk Reduction Counseling in Primary Care to Prevent Sexually Transmitted Infections: An Updated Systematic Evidence Review for the U.S. Preventive Services Task Force

Prepared for:
Agency for Healthcare Research and Quality
U.S. Department of Health and Human Services
540 Gaither Road
Rockville, MD 20850
www.ahrq.gov

Contract No. HHSA-290-2012-00151-I, Task Order No. 2

Prepared by:
Kaiser Permanente Research Affiliates Evidence-based Practice Center
Kaiser Permanente Center for Health Research
Portland, OR

Investigators:
Elizabeth O'Connor, PhD
Jennifer S. Lin, MD, MCR
Brittany U. Burda, MPH
Jillian T. Henderson, PhD
Emily S. Walsh, MPH
Evelyn P. Whitlock, MD, MPH

AHRQ Publication No. 13-05180-EF-1
September 2014

This report is based on research conducted by the Kaiser Permanente Research Affiliates Evidence-based Practice Center (EPC) under contract to the Agency for Healthcare Research and Quality (AHRQ), Rockville, MD (Contract No. HHSA-290-2012-00151-I, Task Order No. 2). The findings and conclusions in this document are those of the authors, who are responsible for its contents, and do not necessarily represent the views of AHRQ. Therefore, no statement in this report should be construed as an official position of AHRQ or of the U.S. Department of Health and Human Services.

The information in this report is intended to help health care decisionmakers—patients and clinicians, health system leaders, and policymakers, among others—make well-informed decisions and thereby improve the quality of health care services. This report is not intended to be a substitute for the application of clinical judgment.

This report may be used, in whole or in part, as the basis for development of clinical practice guidelines and other quality enhancement tools, or as a basis for reimbursement and coverage policies. AHRQ or U.S. Department of Health and Human Services endorsement of such derivative products may not be stated or implied.

This document is in the public domain and may be used and reprinted without permission except those copyrighted materials that are clearly noted in the document. Further reproduction of those copyrighted materials is prohibited without the specific permission of copyright holders.

None of the investigators has any affiliations or financial involvement that conflicts with the material presented in this report.

Acknowledgments

The authors gratefully acknowledge the following individuals for their contributions to this project: Karen Lee, MD, MPH, at AHRQ; current and former members of the U.S. Preventive Services Task Force who contributed to topic deliberations; Ralph J. DiClemente, PhD, for providing expert review; Peter Miele, MD, and the Centers for Disease Control and Prevention for providing federal partner review of the report; and Smyth Lai, MLS, and Kevin Lutz, MFA, at the Kaiser Permanente Center for Health Research.

Suggested Citation

O'Connor E, Lin JS, Burda BU, Henderson JT, Walsh ES, Whitlock EP. Behavioral Sexual Risk Reduction Counseling in Primary Care to Prevent Sexually Transmitted Infections: An Updated Systematic Evidence Review for the U.S. Preventive Services Task Force. Evidence Synthesis No. 114. AHRQ Publication No. 13-05180-EF-1. Rockville, MD: Agency for Healthcare Research and Quality; 2014.

Structured Abstract

Background: Sexually transmitted infections (STIs) are common and a source of substantial morbidity in the United States. Behavioral sexual risk reduction counseling in primary care may help prevent STIs.

Purpose: To systematically review evidence on the benefits and harms of primary care–relevant behavioral counseling interventions designed to reduce STIs through reductions in risky sexual behaviors and increased protective sexual behaviors, to aid the U.S. Preventive Services Task Force (USPSTF) in updating its recommendation on this topic.

Methods: Building on a previous review for the USPSTF, we searched a number of databases, including MEDLINE, PubMed, PsycINFO, and the Cochrane Collaboration Registry of Controlled Trials, to identify relevant literature published since the previous review (January 1, 2007 through November 4, 2012). We also examined references of other existing systematic reviews; searched Web sites of government agencies, professional organizations, and other organizations for grey literature; and monitored health news Web sites and journal tables of contents to identify potentially eligible trials. Two investigators independently reviewed identified abstracts and full-text articles against a set of a priori inclusion and quality criteria. One investigator abstracted data into an evidence table and a second investigator checked these data. We conducted random-effects meta-analyses to estimate the effect of sexual risk reduction counseling on STI incidence and, for adults only, condom use.

Results: We included 31 trials reported in 57 publications; 16 (n=56,110) were newly published trials that were not included in the previous review, and 15 trials (n=14,214) were included in the previous review. High-intensity (>2 hours) interventions reduced STI incidence in adolescents and adults. Low- and moderate-intensity interventions were generally not effective in adults; however, we identified some promising low- and moderate-intensity approaches. Moderate-intensity interventions may be effective in adolescents, but data were sparse. Pooled effects showed the odds of acquiring an STI were reduced by 62 percent in adolescents (k=5) and 30 percent in adults (k=9) with high-intensity interventions. Reported behavioral outcomes were heterogeneous, and results were most likely to show a benefit with high-intensity interventions at 6 months or less. Most trials targeted populations at increased risk for STIs, as defined by sociodemographic characteristics, history of risky sexual behaviors, or history of an STI. We found no evidence that sexual risk reduction counseling could be harmful.

Conclusions: High-intensity behavioral sexual risk reduction counseling can reduce the incidence of STIs in primary care and related clinical settings, especially in sexually active adolescents and in adults at increased risk for STIs. Less intensive interventions may also be effective in adolescents, but these data are still sparse. Findings are consistent with and expand upon the previous review on this topic.

Table of Contents

CHAPTER 1. INTRODUCTION 1
    Condition Definition 1
    Prevalence and Burden 1
        Bacterial Infections.. 1
        Viral Infections... 2
        Parasitic Infections 3
    Etiology and Natural History 4
    Risk Factors 4
    Sexual Health History and Risk Assessment 5
    Counseling Interventions to Prevent STIs 5
    Current Clinical Practice in the United States 6
    Current Initiatives in the United States... 6
    Related USPSTF Recommendations 7
    Previous USPSTF Recommendation 7
CHAPTER 2. METHODS 8
    Scope and Purpose 8
    Key Questions and Analytic Framework 8
    Data Sources and Searches 8
    Study Selection 9
    Quality Assessment and Data Abstraction... 10
    Data Synthesis and Analysis 10
    Expert Review and Public Comment 12
    USPSTF Involvement 12
CHAPTER 3. RESULTS 13
    Literature Search... 13
    Description of Included Studies... 13
    KQ 1. Is There Direct Evidence That Behavioral Counseling Interventions to Reduce Risky Sexual Behaviors and Increase Protective Sexual Behaviors Reduce STI Incidence and/or Related Morbidity and Mortality? 15
        Results in Adolescents.. 16
        Results in Adults 17
    KQ 2. Do Behavioral Counseling Interventions to Prevent STIs Reduce Risky Sexual Behavior or Increase Protective Sexual Behavior? 19
        Results in Adolescents.. 19
        Results in Adults 20
    KQs 1a, 2a. Are There Population or Intervention Characteristics That Influence the Effectiveness of Interventions? 20
        Important Population Characteristics 21
        Important Intervention Characteristics... 24
    KQ 3. Are There Other Positive Outcomes Beside STI Incidence and Changes in Risky or Protective Sexual Behavior From Behavioral Counseling Interventions to Prevent STIs?..... 27
    KQ 4. What Adverse Effects Are Associated With Behavioral Counseling Interventions to Prevent STIs in Primary Care?... 28

CHAPTER 4. DISCUSSION **29**
   Summary of Evidence 29
   Important Components of Sexual Risk Reduction Counseling 30
   Public Health Impact 31
   Acceptability of Sexual Risk Reduction Counseling 32
   Limitations of the Review 34
      Limitations of Our Report 34
      Limitations of the Data on Populations 34
      Limitations of the Data on Other STI Prevention Strategies 35
   Future Research Needs 36
   Conclusion 37
REFERENCES **38**

Figures
Figure 1. Analytic Framework
Figure 2. Included Trials, by Intervention Intensity and Population Risk, Showing the Primary Outcome and Noting Trials With Narrowly Targeted Samples
Figure 3. Distribution of Included Studies Across the Levels of Treatment Intensity and Population Risk, Weighted by Sample Size
Figure 4. Forest Plot of STI Incidence in Included Trials Targeting Adolescents
Figure 5. Forest Plot of STI Incidence in Included Trials Targeting Adults
Figure 6. Forest Plot of Condom Use and Unprotected Sexual Intercourse in Included Trials Targeting Adults

Tables
Table 1. Recommendations of Other Organizations for Sexual Risk Reduction Counseling to Prevent STIs
Table 2. Design and Baseline Population Characteristics of Included Studies Targeting Adolescents
Table 3. Design and Baseline Population Characteristics of Included Studies Targeting Adults
Table 4. Summary of Included Studies—Adolescents
Table 5. Summary of Included Studies—Adults
Table 6. Summary of Evidence
Table 7. Estimated Number Needed to Treat to Prevent One STI and the Number of Fewer STIs per 1,000 Persons With Sexual Risk Reduction Counseling

Appendixes
Appendix A. Detailed Methods
Appendix B. Excluded Studies
Appendix C. Summary Tables
Appendix D. Ongoing Studies

CHAPTER 1. INTRODUCTION

Condition Definition

Sexually transmitted infections (STIs) are infections that are primarily transmitted through sexual contact (e.g., vaginal, anal, or oral intercourse).[1] The STIs with the most substantial public health impact in the United States include human immunodeficiency virus (HIV), hepatitis B virus infection (HBV), herpes simplex virus (HSV) 1 and 2, human papillomavirus (HPV), *Chlamydia trachomatis*, *Neisseria gonorrhea*, *Treponema pallidum* (syphilis), and *Trichomonas vaginalis*. Other STIs include bacterial vaginosis (BV), granuloma inguinale, chancroid, pubic lice, and *Sarcoptes scabiei* var. *hominis* (scabies).

Prevalence and Burden

The Centers for Disease Control (CDC) estimate that approximately 20 million new cases of STIs occur each year in the United States and more than two thirds of those cases are among persons ages 15 to 24 years.[2] Point prevalence for any of the five most common STIs among females ages 14 to 19 was 24 percent in 2003 to 2004, and 38 percent among those who were sexually active.[3] In 2010, the inflation-adjusted annual direct medical costs of STIs (including HIV) were $16.9 billion in the United States.[4]

Bacterial Infections

Chlamydia

In 2011, 1,412,791 cases of *Chlamydia trachomatis* infection were reported to the CDC. This represents the largest number of cases ever reported to the CDC for any condition and is an 8 percent increase from the rate in 2010. This rate reflects an overall rate in U.S. women (648.9 cases per 100,000 females) that is more than 2.5 times greater than the rate in men (256.9 cases per 100,000 males). In 2011, the age-specific rates of chlamydia in women were highest among those ages 15 to 19 years (3,416.5 cases per 100,000 females) and 20 to 24 years (3,722.5 cases per 100,000 females). In 2011, age-specific rates in men were highest among those ages 20 to 24 years (1,343.3 cases per 100,000 males).[5]

Chlamydial infections can result in pelvic inflammatory disease (PID) in women, which is a major cause of infertility, ectopic pregnancy, and chronic pelvic pain. Chlamydial infection can also facilitate HIV transmission. Pregnant women infected with chlamydia can transmit the infection during delivery, which can result in neonatal ophthalmia and pneumonia.[5]

Gonorrhea

In 2011, 321,849 cases of gonorrhea were reported in the United States (104.2 cases per 100,000 population), with the highest rates occurring in the southern United States. Gonorrhea rates were slightly higher among women (108.9 cases per 100,000) than men (98.7 cases per 100,000). In 2011, gonorrhea rates were highest among females ages 20 to 24 years (584.2 cases per 100,000) and 15 to 19 years (556.5 cases per 100,000). In men, the rate of gonorrhea was highest among those ages 20 to 24 years (450.6 cases per 100,000).

Gonococcal infections, like chlamydial infections, can cause PID in women. Treating gonorrhea is complicated by antimicrobial resistance in the United States, as the only class of antibiotics recommended for the treatment of gonorrhea is cephalosporins.[5]

Syphilis

In 2011, the overall reported cases of primary and secondary syphilis in the United States was 13,970. Primary and secondary syphilis rates are higher among men (8.2 cases per 100,000) than women (1.0 case per 100,000). Syphilis rates are highest among adults ages 20 to 24 years (13.8 cases per 100,000) and 25 to 29 years (12.1 cases per 100,000).

As with chlamydia, syphilis facilitates the transmission of HIV infection. If untreated, early syphilis in pregnant women results in perinatal death in up to 40 percent of cases. If acquired during the 4 years prior to pregnancy, untreated syphilis can lead to infection of the fetus in 80 percent of cases. Transmission of syphilis to the fetus during pregnancy can result in fetal death or an infant born with physical and mental developmental disabilities. The rate of congenital syphilis was 8.7 cases per 100,000 live births in 2010.[5] This rate represented a decrease since 2008 (from 10.5 cases per 100,000 live births).

Viral Infections

HIV

About 1.2 million people in the United States are living with HIV infection, and one in five are unaware of their infection. Since the HIV epidemic began, an estimated 1,129,127 persons in the United States have been diagnosed with acquired immunodeficiency syndrome (AIDS) and 619,400 have died.[6] In 2009, the estimated rate of HIV diagnoses in the 40 states with confidential name-based reporting systems was 17.4 per 100,000 persons. In 2009, adults ages 20 to 24 years represented the highest rate of diagnoses (36.9 per 100,000 population). African Americans accounted for 52 percent of all diagnoses of HIV infection and males accounted for 76 percent among adults and adolescents. In 2009, most new infections were attributed to sexual contact, either male-to-male (57%) or heterosexual contact (31%).[7] Persons with other STIs have increased risk for transmission and acquisition of HIV. Persons with current STIs are at least 2 to 5 times more likely than uninfected persons to acquire HIV if exposed through sexual contact. Additionally, persons with HIV infection who are also infected with other STIs are more likely to transmit HIV through sexual contact than those who are not infected with other STIs.[8]

The rate of HIV transmission has declined by an estimated 89 percent since the mid-1980s, attributable to HIV prevention efforts, which have saved an estimated $125 billion in medical costs.[9]

HPV

HPV is a common STI. Researchers have estimated that at least 50 percent of sexually active persons will acquire an HPV infection in their lifetime.[1] Data from 2003 to 2005 indicate an overall prevalence of 23 percent for high-risk HPV (types 16, 18, 31, 33, 35, 39, 45, 51, 52, 56, 58, 59, and 68) in the United States. HPV prevalence was highest in females ages 14 to 19 years (35%) and 20 to 29 years (29%).[5] Persistent infection with high-risk HPV can lead to the development of cervical cancer as well as other anogenital and throat cancers. Other HPV strains are associated with genital warts. Although HPV vaccines do exist, HPV is not treatable once acquired. Many women have transitory infections that are spontaneously cleared by the immune system.

HSV 1 and 2

Between 2005 and 2008, 16.2 percent of persons in the United States ages 14 to 49 years had an HSV-2 infection. The overall prevalence of genital herpes, however, is likely higher because an increasing number of genital herpes infections are caused by HSV-1.[10] HSV-2 infection is more prevalent among women (20.9% in females ages 14 to 49 years) than men (11.5% in males ages 14 to 49 years). Most persons with HSV-1 or HSV-2 infection are asymptomatic or have very mild symptoms that may go unnoticed or are mistaken for another skin condition. Nearly 82 percent of persons with HSV-1 or HSV-2 are unaware of their infection. Genital herpes can cause painful ulcers on the genitals that can be particularly severe and persistent in persons with suppressed immune systems. These lesions may also appear in the buttocks, groin, thighs, fingers, and eyes during the course of infection. Persons with genital herpes have an estimated 2- to 4-fold increased risk for acquiring HIV if exposed to that infection. Pregnant women can transmit herpes infection to their child, which can result in a potentially fatal infection in the offspring (neonatal herpes). The risk for perinatal transmission is higher during the first outbreak of symptoms (e.g., blisters) than during a recurrent outbreak. Rarely, HSV-1 and HSV-2 can also cause blindness, encephalitis, and aseptic meningitis.[11]

HBV

In the United States, between 4.3 and 5.6 percent of the population has been infected with HBV at some point during their lives. Between 800,000 and 1.4 million persons in the United States are living with a chronic HBV infection. From 2004 to 2009, the annual number of chronic liver disease deaths associated with HBV was 3,000. In 2009, the estimated total number of new HBV infections was 38,000.[12] The proportion of reported cases attributed to sexual contact is unknown.[13] Effective HBV vaccines have been available in the United States since 1981.[13]

Parasitic Infections

Trichomoniasis

An estimated 3.7 million persons in the United States have a trichomoniasis infection. Trichomoniasis infection is more common in women than men. The prevalence of *Trichomonas vaginalis* infection in the United States is estimated to be 2.3 million (3.1%) among females ages

14 to 49 years. This estimate is based on a sample of women who participated in the National Health and Nutrition Examination Survey from 2001 to 2004. Only about 30 percent of persons with the infection develop any symptoms. Untreated trichomoniasis can cause genital inflammation that facilitates HIV infection or transmission. Pregnant women with trichomoniasis are more likely to have preterm delivery, and babies born to these women are more likely to have low birth weight. Pregnant women represent 3.2 percent of all infections.[14]

Etiology and Natural History

According to 2006 to 2012 data from the National Survey of Family Growth, the average age at first vaginal heterosexual intercourse for women and men was 17.1 years.[15,16] In another study using data from 2007 to 2012, 66 percent of men and women experienced their first oral sexual encounter between the ages of 15 and 24 years.[17] Initiation of oral sex commonly occurs before first vaginal sexual intercourse. According to the National Longitudinal Study of Adolescent Health, younger age at first intercourse is associated with higher odds of STI infection compared with older ages at first intercourse.[18]

While the time from sexual initiation to first STI diagnosis has not been widely studied, one cohort study of 386 adolescent females ages 14 to 17 years who initiated first sexual intercourse at an average age of 14.2 years found that diagnosis of the first STI occurred a median of 2 years after first intercourse.[19] The median time to reinfection was 1.2 years.

While some infected persons may experience no symptoms of the STI, they are still infectious. For example, nearly 70 percent of men and women with a gonococcal or chlamydial infection experience no symptoms.[20] Untreated STIs can lead to serious adverse health outcomes (e.g., infertility, PID, reinfection). Reinfection is also common, especially with gonorrhea, chlamydia, and trichomoniasis. A 2007 systematic review of repeat gonococcal and chlamydial infection among males reported a median rate of reinfection within 12 months of initial diagnosis of 11.3 and 7.0 percent, respectively.[21] A companion 2009 systematic review among females reported a median rate of reinfection within 12 months of initial diagnosis of 13.9 and 11.7 percent, respectively.[22]

The incubation and latency periods between infection, first symptoms, and serious sequelae varies by STI and specific health outcome. The incubation period of gonococcal infection to first symptoms, for example, can be as short as 2 days after exposure. Acute hepatitis can occur within 4 to 24 weeks after HBV exposure. The latency period from HPV infection to manifestation into a precancerous lesion of the cervix, on the other hand, may take as long as 20 years. Since there is no cure for some STIs, prevention and early treatment are critical to averting individual- and population-level adverse health outcomes and spread of disease.

Risk Factors

Risky sexual behaviors can include inconsistent or improper use of barrier contraception, high number of lifetime sex partners, multiple sex partners, sexual intercourse under the influence of mind-altering substances, and sexual intercourse with a partner who has an STI or is at high risk for an STI.

Incidence and prevalence of STIs are elevated in a number of populations in the United States, which increases the risk for exposure. African Americans have the highest risk for STI infection of all racial/ethnic groups. For example, incidence rates of STIs tracked by the CDC are consistently 8 or more times higher in African Americans than whites,[23] and African American youth accounted for 57 percent of all new HIV infections among persons ages 13 to 24 years in 2009.[24] Other racial/ethnic groups with a high prevalence of STIs are American Indians/Alaska Natives and Hispanics.[23] Young persons (age <25 years) are also at higher risk for STIs than those age 25 years or older.[23] STI incidence also varies by region within the United States, with highest rates in the southeast and Alaska.[23] Other populations with high STI rates include men who have sex with men (MSM),[25] persons with low income living in urban settings,[26] military recruits,[27] persons with mental illness or disability,[28] current or former inmates,[29] current or former intravenous drug users,[30] persons with a history of sexual abuse,[31] and persons engaging in transactional sex.[32,33]

While most STIs occur in young adults, there is growing concern about STIs in older adults, as recent epidemiological studies show sharp increases in STI rates among those age 50 years or older.[34] According to 2008 CDC data, 15 percent of new HIV diagnoses occurred in persons age 50 years or older.[35] In another study, also based on CDC data, the rates of syphilis and chlamydia increased 43 percent from 2005 to 2009 in adults age 55 years or older.[36] The increase in STI rates among adults age 50 years or older may be attributable to limited sexual health services, increased longevity, and the availability of sexual performance enhancement drugs.[34]

Sexual Health History and Risk Assessment

Primary care physicians have an opportunity to assess a patient's risk for acquiring STIs during the patient visit. A comprehensive sexual health history assesses the patient's sexual activity and other related behaviors that increase their risk for an STI and becoming pregnant.[37] Important items in a sexual health history include sexual orientation (i.e., sexual preference), frequency of sexual activity and the number of partners, and type of sexual engagement (e.g., penile-vaginal intercourse, oral sex, anal sex).[37] Several national organizations, including the American Academy of Pediatrics, the American Academy of Family Physicians, the American Congress of Obstetrics and Gynecology, the Society for Adolescent Health and Medicine, the American Medical Association, and the Institute of Medicine recommend that physicians periodically obtain a sexual history or sexual risk assessment and discuss risk reduction with all patients. Many of the aforementioned professional organizations have developed sexual history taking or sexual risk assessment tools for providers to use in primary care.

Counseling Interventions to Prevent STIs

The CDC recommends that health care providers inform patients on how to reduce their risk for STI transmission, including abstinence, correct and consistent condom use, and limiting the number of sex partners. It recommends an interactive, empathic, and nonjudgmental approach that is tailored to the patient's personal risk, with personalized goal setting.[1] The CDC maintains a Web site of interventions it considers effective for HIV risk reduction, including more than 25 behavioral interventions tailored for a variety of different populations.[38] These interventions commonly include motivational and cognitive behavioral elements, such as goal setting, skills development with role play, communication or negotiation training, values clarification exercises, and problem solving.

Current Clinical Practice in the United States

Representative surveys examining STI counseling practices among U.S. physicians have varied findings. In a survey of 508 pediatricians, for example, only 28 percent offered sexual risk reduction guidance to the parents of their adolescent patients.[39] In another survey conducted among 1,217 Californian internists, family physicians, obstetricians-gynecologists, and pediatricians, 31 percent reported educating their adolescent patients about STI/HIV transmission and 36 percent reported educating their sexually active adolescent patients.[40] Among 541 surveyed Pennsylvania primary care physicians, 88% reported asking their adolescent and young adult patients (ages 15 to 25 years) about sexual activity and 80 percent reported counseling those patients about STI/HIV transmission and prevention.[41] In the same study, however, 70 percent of physicians believed STI counseling in general to be ineffective. Primary care physicians frequently reported insufficient time as the main barrier to providing STI and/or HIV counseling during a patient visit.[41-45] National data from the Youth Adult Health Care Survey indicate that nearly half of adolescents reported that they did not receive guidance on various age-appropriate topics, including sexual activity, contraception, and STIs, during their previous health examination.[46]

Rates of STI counseling are higher among physicians working in STI clinics—81 percent reported counseling and 25 percent specifically developed a risk reduction plan with the patient.[47]

Current Initiatives in the United States

In 2001, the U.S. Surgeon General issued a call to action to promote sexual health and responsible sexual behavior.[48] These strategies included increasing awareness, implementing and strengthening interventions, and expanding the research base relating to sexual health matters. In 2007, the CDC Division of STD Prevention released a strategic plan to provide national leadership, research, policy development, and scientific information to help Americans live safer, healthier lives through the prevention of STIs and their complications.[49] The seven strategic goals included:

- Preventing STI-related infertility
- Preventing STI-related adverse outcomes of pregnancy
- Preventing STI-related cancers
- Preventing STI-related HIV transmission

- Strengthening STI prevention capacity and infrastructure
- Reducing STI health disparities across and within communities and populations
- Addressing the effects of the social and economic determinants and costs of specific STIs and associated sequelae among specific populations.

Currently, the CDC has two initiatives to inform the public and reduce or eliminate STIs: the Syphilis Elimination Effort and the Infertility and Prevention Project, which promotes screening for chlamydia and gonorrhea.[50] The Healthy People 2020 initiative[51] has published 10 goals related to reducing the proportion of adolescents and young adults with chlamydia, gonorrhea, syphilis, HPV, and HSV-2.

Recommendations from other health organizations for STI counseling in clinical practice are listed in **Table 1**.

Related U.S. Preventive Services Task Force Recommendations

The U.S. Preventive Services Task Force (USPSTF) has issued several recommendations related to screening for STIs. While specific details vary, the USPSTF generally recommends that primary care physicians: 1) screen sexually active, nonpregnant women at increased risk for STIs for chlamydia, gonorrhea, HIV, and syphilis; 2) screen all pregnant women for HBV, HIV, and syphilis and screen pregnant women at increased risk for STIs for chlamydia and gonorrhea; 3) screen all men for HIV and screen sexually active men at increased risk for STIs for syphilis; and 4) do not screen men and women who are not at increased risk for STIs, except for HIV.[52]

Previous USPSTF Recommendation

In 2008, the USPSTF concluded there was moderate certainty that high-intensity behavioral counseling interventions targeted to sexually active adolescents and adults at increased risk for STIs have a moderate net benefit on the incidence of STIs. Therefore, the USPSTF recommended high-intensity behavioral counseling for all sexually active adolescents and for adults at increased risk for STIs (B recommendation). The evidence was insufficient to assess the balance of benefits and harms of behavioral counseling to prevent STIs in nonsexually active adolescents and in adults not at increased risk for STIs (I statement).

CHAPTER 2. METHODS

Scope and Purpose

This systematic review addresses the benefits and harms of behavioral sexual risk reduction counseling interventions in primary care to prevent STIs among adolescents and adults. The USPSTF will use this review to update its 2008 recommendation on behavioral counseling to prevent STIs.[53]

Key Questions and Analytic Framework

We developed an analytic framework (**Figure 1**) and four Key Questions (KQs) to guide our review, in consultation with the Agency for Healthcare Research and Quality (AHRQ) and members of the USPSTF. These KQs were adapted from the questions addressed in the 2008 review.[54]

1. Is there direct evidence that behavioral counseling interventions to reduce risky sexual behaviors and increase protective sexual behaviors reduce STI incidence and/or related morbidity and mortality?
   a. Are there populations or intervention characteristics that influence the effectiveness of the interventions?
2. Do behavioral counseling interventions to prevent STIs reduce risky sexual behavior or increase protective sexual behavior?
   a. Are there populations or intervention characteristics that influence the effectiveness of the interventions?
3. Are there other positive outcomes beside STI incidence and changes in risky or protective sexual behavior from behavioral counseling interventions to prevent STIs?
4. What adverse effects are associated with behavioral counseling interventions to prevent STIs in primary care?

Data Sources and Searches

We performed comprehensive literature searches in the following databases: PubMed, Database of Abstracts of Reviews of Effects, Cochrane Database of Systematic Reviews, British Medical Journal Clinical Evidence, Institute of Medicine, National Institute for Health and Care Excellence, MEDLINE, PsycINFO, Cochrane Central Register of Controlled Trials, and the Cumulative Index to Nursing and Allied Health from January 1, 2007 through November 4, 2013. Our research librarian designed this literature search to identify studies published since the 2008 review (**Appendix A**). We limited all searches to articles published in the English language. We managed literature search results using Reference Manager® version 12.0 (Thomson Reuters, New York, NY).

We also reviewed reference lists of included studies and relevant reviews and meta-analyses to identify potentially relevant studies that were published prior to our literature search dates or not identified in our literature searches. We obtained additional references from expert reviewers, members of the public, and bibliographies of other sources (e.g., clinical guidelines). We conducted grey literature searches of government agencies, professional organizations, and other organizations that may sponsor or publish relevant research. We also supplemented our searches with articles identified through news and table-of-contents alerts from Google (Google, Inc., Mountain View, CA), ScienceDirect (Elsevier B.V., Maryland Heights, MO), and HighWire Press (Stanford University Libraries, Palo Alto, CA).

Study Selection

Two investigators independently reviewed titles and abstracts. Investigators then reviewed the full-text articles against prespecified inclusion and exclusion criteria (**Appendix A Table 1**). Disagreements were resolved through discussion and consensus.

We included randomized, controlled trials and nonrandomized, controlled clinical trials with interventions targeting risky sexual behaviors to prevent STIs (alone or in combination with other behaviors) in adults and adolescents, including pregnant women, of any sexual orientation or level of sexual activity. We excluded studies limited to persons who were HIV positive or populations that had very high HIV prevalence, inmates and court-involved persons, and psychiatric inpatients (i.e., ≥50% of the study population was institutionalized or in supportive housing). Although these patient populations are seen in primary care, trials aimed at these populations were excluded from this review because their results may not be generalizable to general primary care populations, and the results of these trials do not help inform the question of whether counseling should be routinely offered in primary care settings.

We excluded studies that exclusively targeted unintended pregnancy or another behavior (e.g., drug use) associated with risky sexual behavior without directly addressing STI prevention in the intervention, even if they reported relevant biological or behavioral outcomes. We also excluded studies without control groups. Control groups could include usual care, attention control, minimal intervention (≤15 minutes), wait list, or no intervention.

Included studies had to be conducted in or recruited from primary care, mental health clinics, reproductive health clinics (including STI clinics), or from broader health care systems in developed countries (with "very high" human development according to the World Health Organization).[55] We excluded studies in worksites, schools (except school health clinics), or other settings that were not generalizable to primary care. We also excluded studies with interventions that included components that could not be implemented in primary care settings, such as communitywide media messages or interventions conducted within existing social networks (e.g., churches, social clubs).

We included studies that reported health outcomes (STI incidence or related morbidity), behavioral outcomes (changes in sexual behavior), or adverse effects of sexual risk reduction counseling (e.g., care avoidance, shame, guilt, stigma). Any additional reported outcomes that could be related to harms were also abstracted from studies meeting inclusion criteria (e.g., stress, acceptability ratings). Similarly, other positive outcomes (e.g., reductions in unintended pregnancy) were also abstracted, but were not sufficient to warrant inclusion in the review. We required at least 3 months postbaseline followup for all outcomes except harms.

Consistent with the 2008 review, we excluded trials published before 1988, as these were largely conducted before HIV/AIDS was identified and current approaches to medical management were developed.

Quality Assessment and Data Abstraction

Two investigators independently assessed the quality of included studies using predefined criteria from the USPSTF[56] and assigned each a final quality rating of "good," "fair," or "poor" (**Appendix A Table 2**). Investigators resolved disagreements through discussion. We excluded studies rated as poor quality (i.e., attrition >40%, differential attrition >20%, other "fatal flaws," or the cumulative effects of multiple minor flaws or missing enough important information to limit our confidence in the validity of the results) (**Appendix B**). Good-quality studies had adequate randomization procedures, allocation concealment, blinding of outcome assessors, reliable outcome measures, comparable groups at baseline (with specified eligibility criteria) and followup, low attrition, acceptable statistical methods, and adequate and faithful adherence to the intervention. In addition, we also considered whether the study evaluated a biological outcome. We rated studies as fair quality if they did not meet most of the good-quality criteria.

One investigator abstracted data from all included studies into a standard evidence table and a second investigator checked the data for accuracy. We abstracted study design characteristics, population demographics, baseline sexual history, intervention details, biological outcomes, behavioral outcomes (e.g., condom use, sex partners, unprotected sex, and other sexual activity), other positive outcomes (e.g., reduction in unintended pregnancy), and adverse events.

Data Synthesis and Analysis

We created separate tables for the results for each KQ and created additional summary tables of key trial characteristics and results. We qualitatively examined these tables to identify the range of results and potential associations with effect size. We examined trials that targeted only adolescents separately from those that targeted adults (some of which also included adolescents). We also examined subgroup analyses limited to adolescents from three trials with a wide age range.[57-59] Because we planned a priori to present data separately for adolescents and adults in our report, we abstracted age-specific results when they were presented, even if there was no indication in the trial methods that subgroup analyses by age were planned a priori. We analyzed adolescents separately because the developmental differences between adolescents and adults may warrant different intervention approaches and targets (e.g., delayed sexual debut or reduced sexual activity may be appropriate only for adolescents).

Within age strata, we further stratified tables by intervention intensity: low (single session, estimated ≤30 minutes of intervention contact), moderate (30 to 120 minutes of intervention contact), or high (>2 hours of intervention contact). We also categorized studies into one of four risk strata: 1) mixture of sexually active and presexually active participants (relevant for adolescents only); 2) sexually active participants with no further risk factors required and not in an increased-risk setting (relevant for adults only); 3) participants with increased risk based on characteristics of the population (e.g., adolescents, low-income inner-city residents, African Americans, Latinos, American Indians/Alaska Natives, MSM, military recruits, persons with mental illness or disability, intravenous drug users, persons with a history of sexual abuse, sex workers, or persons reporting high-risk behaviors) or setting (e.g., STI clinics, clinics in low-income inner-city locations, or clinics serving a high proportion of patients at increased risk); and 4) persons at high risk based on a current or recent STI. Within risk strata, we grouped studies by setting (primary care, reproductive health clinic, STI clinic, other setting).

We conducted random-effects meta-analyses for STI incidence using the DerSimonian and Laird method, with separate pooling for adolescents and adults. Because some of our pooled estimates were derived from combining a small number of trials, we ran sensitivity analyses using the profile likelihood method, which is more conservative when the number of studies is small. All statistically significant results remained within the profile likelihood method. Results shown are those using the DerSimonian and Laird method.

We used Stata 11.2 (StataCorp LP, College Station, TX) for all statistical analysis. We analyzed odds ratios (ORs) based on reported adjusted ORs if available. We used unadjusted ORs if adjusted results were not available. We used the raw numbers of events and numbers of participants with followup if ORs were not available. For condom use outcomes, we included any measure of the proportion using condoms by group, including use at most recent intercourse, consistent use, and any use. If a trial reported the proportion reporting any unprotected sex, we subtracted the number from 100 percent and included those data in the condom use analysis.

We stratified our primary analysis by intervention intensity. If trials included more than one treatment arm and these arms fell into different intensity categories, we included both treatment arms but only pooled within the intensity categories. As such, trials never contributed more than one data point to a pooled estimate. If there were multiple intervention arms within the same intensity category, we included the arm that was most intensive or comprehensive in the meta-analysis.

We assessed the presence of statistical heterogeneity among the studies using standard chi-squared tests and estimated the magnitude of heterogeneity using the I^2 statistic.[60] We applied the Cochrane Collaboration's rules of thumb for interpreting heterogeneity: less than 40 percent likely represents unimportant heterogeneity, 30 to 65 percent represents moderate heterogeneity, 50 to 90 percent represents substantial heterogeneity, and greater than 75 percent indicates considerable heterogeneity.[61] We also included prediction intervals in forest plots, which provide an estimate of where 95 percent of newly conducted trials would fall, assuming the between-study variability in the included trials held for new trials.[62] Prediction intervals are shown with pooled estimates on forest plots, and the horizontal lines represent the 95 percent confidence interval (CI) of the pooled effect.

We examined small-study effects on STI outcomes using funnel plots, Peter's test for small-study effects, and Harbord's modified test for small-study effects, combining adult and adolescent trials. These tests examined whether the distribution of the effect sizes was symmetric with respect to effect precision. The results of these tests were contradictory; Peter's test suggested the presence of small-study effects, while Harbord's did not. Visual inspection of the funnel plot showed that two trials with large effects and few events seemed to be driving asymmetry in the funnel plot.[63,64] We tested this hypothesis by excluding these two trials and re-running the two tests of small-study effects. After excluding these studies, neither test indicated the presence of small-study effects. One of these trials was the only low-intensity trial in adolescents, so it was not combined with other trials in the meta-analysis and therefore does not put pooled estimates at risk for bias. The other trial was a high-intensity trial in adults, which had the smallest weight of all high-intensity trials in the meta-analysis. Therefore, we believe that the pooled effect estimate is no more than minimally biased by small-study effects, because of this study's small contribution to the pooled effect.

We calculated the number needed to treat (NNT) to prevent one STI and the number of cases prevented based on the pooled OR at three levels of baseline risk.[61] For baseline risk, we chose incidence rates of 5, 15, and 25 percent. This same process was used to estimate CIs for the NNTs, using the CIs of the pooled ORs.

Expert Review and Public Comment

A draft research plan for this topic was available for public comment from January 29 to February 25, 2013. The draft version of this report was reviewed by experts and USPSTF federal partners and posted for public comment on the USPSTF Web site from April 29 to May 26, 2014. No new substantive issues were identified that were not previously considered, and no major changes were made to the final report. Comments received during any period were reviewed, considered, and addressed as appropriate.

USPSTF Involvement

This research was funded by AHRQ under a contract to support the USPSTF. We consulted with four USPSTF liaisons at key points in the review, including the development of the research plan (i.e., KQs, analytic framework, and inclusion/exclusion criteria), as well as finalizing the systematic review. An AHRQ Medical Officer provided project oversight, reviewed the draft and final versions of the report, and assisted with public comment on the research plan and draft evidence report. The USPSTF and AHRQ had no role in the study selection, quality assessment, or writing of the systematic review.

CHAPTER 3. RESULTS

Literature Search

We included 31 trials in the review.[57-59,63-90] The results of these trials were reported in 57 publications and were selected from our review of 3,241 abstracts and 218 full-text articles (**Appendix A Figure 1**). We identified 23 trials examining the primary effects of behavioral counseling interventions on health outcomes;[57-59,63,64,67-74,78-80,83-85,87-90] 25 trials examined the effects on sexual behaviors;[57-59,63-68,71-73,75-77,79,81-88,90] nine trials examined the effects on other positive outcomes;[59,63,66,68,70-72,75,81] and only three trials reported on adverse effects of the intervention.[84,85,90]

Description of Included Studies

Of the 31 included trials (n=70,324), 16 were newly published trials that were not included in the previous review (n=56,110) and 15 were included in the 2008 review (n=14,214). **Figure 2** lists all included studies stratified by intervention intensity and population risk. The majority of the trials targeted participants at increased risk for STIs or with a recent STI, and most trials provided high-intensity interventions. **Figure 3** shows the distribution of trials across the levels of treatment intensity and population risk, weighted by sample size. Notably, three newly added trials provided low-intensity interventions to participants at increased risk, including one large trial conducted in STI clinics.[78]

Tables 2 to 5 provide information about the study samples, intervention characteristics, and outcomes reported, organized by intervention intensity, with separate tables for adolescents and adults. Trials that conducted subgroup analyses by age are shown in both adolescent and adult tables. Detailed intervention descriptions are in **Appendix C Table 1**.

Nine trials examined outcomes in adolescents. Six of these trials were limited to adolescents,[63,65-69] and three additional trials included a wide age range, but reported subgroup analyses limited to adolescents.[57-59] Twenty-five trials examined outcomes in adults, including trials covering both adolescents and adults.[57-59,64,70-90] Most of the adult trials either targeted young adults (age <25 years) or had an average age of 25 years or younger, so adults older than age 30 years are only minimally represented, and adults older than age 50 years are represented even less.

According to our risk categorization, eight trials were in the highest risk category, which required a current or recent STI for inclusion.[57,69,73,74,85-88] Sixteen trials included participants with elevated risk, primarily based on sociodemographic characteristics of the population or setting.[58,59,64,67,68,71,72,78-84,89,90] Four included trials recruited sexually active persons primarily from adult populations with no further risk factors required and not in high-risk settings.[70,75-77] Finally, three trials limited their populations to adolescents and included both sexually and nonsexually active youth.[63,65,66]

Seventeen of the trials included only women and three included only men. The remaining trial populations ranged from 30 to 72 percent female. Excluding the large (n=40,282) trial by Warner and colleagues[78] (which only included 30% females), an estimated 62 percent of included participants were female. In 19 of the trials, greater than 75 percent of the participants were African American and/or Latino, including 11 trials exclusively in persons of African American and/or Latino descent. After excluding the large Warner trial[78] (in which 54% of participants were nonwhite), an estimated 77 percent of participants were nonwhite and primarily African American or Latino. None of the included trials targeted MSM, and only two trials included a sizeable proportion of MSM.[78,90] Both of these trials reported results separately for MSM and heterosexual men. One other trial targeted women who have sex with women and have BV to reduce subsequent infection by increasing condom use for digital-vaginal intercourse and on shared insertive sex toys.[74]

All interventions sought to minimize high-risk sexual behaviors (e.g., unprotected sexual intercourse, multiple partners, sex while intoxicated) and maximize protective behaviors (e.g., consistent correct condom use). Interventions provided at least basic information about STIs, such as prevalence and how to prevent transmission. Interventions had a variety of theoretical underpinnings, including the AIDS Risk Reduction Model (ARRM);[57,69,73,81,88] social cognitive theory;[58,59,68,75,79,89] Information, Motivation, Behavior, Skills Model (IMB);[64,87] transtheoretical model;[72,84] health belief model;[71] theory of reasoned action;[58] theory of gender and power;[89] and the model of client health behavior.[85] In addition to basic education, interventions commonly included an individualized risk assessment (self-assessment or assessed by the interventionist), hands-on skills training in condom use, problem solving, decisionmaking, goal setting, and communication about condom use and safe sex, often including role playing. Three additional trials addressed broader relationship issues, such as discussions about what participants believe is important in a relationship.[57,69,81] Techniques to increase motivation to practice safe sex were commonly used, including motivational interviewing. Three trials included HIV testing as part of their interventions.[58,77,90] Many interventions were extensively culturally tailored to a target group, usually based on age, gender, and/or ethnicity. Examples include the trial by DiClemente and colleagues,[68] Sister-to-Sister: The Black Women's Health Project,[79] and Mano a Mano-Mujer,[75] among others.[57,67,69,73,87,89] Four trials targeted prevention of unintended pregnancy as well as STI transmission.[66,70-72] One Spanish trial was limited to women with genital warts and included treatment of their lesions as part of the intervention.[86]

Interventions included between one and 13 sessions, with multiple-session interventions generally lasting 3 months or less. One third of the included trials involved only a single session, including some that were moderate- and high-intensity because of the length of the session. Two additional trials included treatment arms with only one brief session as well as more intensive treatment arms.[79,84] Only two interventions involved continued contact for longer than 5 months and both employed lower-intensity booster contacts after the completion of the main intervention.[82,85] Most of the high-intensity interventions involved group sessions, and some included these group sessions in addition to individual counseling sessions.[69,73,84,85] Most of the low-intensity interventions involved individual meetings with a counselor, but three involved only mail-,[83] computer-,[72] or video-based[78] interventions.

Almost all (28/31 or 90%) of the trials were conducted in the United States. The most common settings were primary care (15/31 or 48%), STI clinics (8/31 or 26%), and other reproductive health clinics, such as obstetrics/gynecology or Planned Parenthood clinics (3/31 or 10%). Only four of the interventions involved the participant's primary care provider or gynecologist in the delivery of the intervention, including two of the three trials conducted outside the United States. Other types of interventionists included health educators, nurses, nurse practitioners, trained lay educators, and other trained facilitators with educational backgrounds ranging from a bachelor's to a medical degree.

Most trials included usual care, a minimal intervention, or waitlist controls. Nine of the trials, however, used attention-control conditions that provided interventions on other healthy lifestyle topics or on topics targeted to the population (e.g., prenatal classes in the trial of pregnant women[59]).

We rated seven of the 31 trials as good quality.[67,68,78,81,82,89,90] We rated the remaining trials as fair quality. We rated 13 additional trials as poor quality and excluded them from the review.[91-103] The most common reasons these trials were rated as poor quality were high (>40%) attrition or substantial differences between groups at baseline. Sixty-one percent of the included trials reported valid randomization procedures and 61 percent reported allocation concealment. Forty-two percent of these trials reported blinding of outcomes assessment, although some trials that did not report outcomes assessment blinding relied on computer- or self-administered questionnaires, so they may not have been adversely affected by lack of blinding. Followup in the included trials ranged from 60 to 97 percent. One trial had high attrition at all followups beyond the initial 3-month followup, so those data were not included.[85] Only six trials reported followup for greater than 90 percent of participants at one or more followups,[63,65,73,74,78,81] and eight had overall followup of less than 80 percent at one or more followups (**Appendix C Tables 11 and 12**).[58,69,72,84,85,87-89]

KQ 1. Is There Direct Evidence That Behavioral Counseling Interventions to Reduce Risky Sexual Behaviors and Increase Protective Sexual Behaviors Reduce STI Incidence and/or Related Morbidity and Mortality?

Twenty-three of the trials reported an STI outcome (n=66,902) (**Appendix C Tables 3** and **4**),[57-59,63,64,67-74,78-80,83-85,87-90] and 20 of these were included in the meta-analysis.[57-59,63,64,67-69,71-73,78-80,83,85,87-90] Ten of these trials were conducted in or recruited from primary care.[59,63,67,68,70,72,79,83,85,89] STI results were generally based on laboratory tests, most commonly for gonorrhea and chlamydia. The next most common STIs assessed were trichomoniasis, syphilis, and HIV, and some trials also included additional infections (e.g., HSV, HPV, granuloma inguinale, lymphogranuloma venereum). One trial focused exclusively on BV prevention in women who have sex with women.[74]

Some trials collected their own laboratory specimens, while other trials supplemented their own specimen results with information from medical records or relied solely on medical records for laboratory test results. While some trials clearly detailed their approach to specimen collection, other trials did not clearly articulate whether specimens were collected for study purposes or clinical uses. Three trials were limited to self-reported STI information.[63,64,83]

Results in Adolescents

Seven trials with eight treatment arms (n=3,407) reported STI outcomes in adolescent populations (**Table 4**). While five of these trials included high-intensity interventions (one of which also included a moderate-intensity arm),[57,58,67-69] one trial had a moderate-intensity arm[59] and another had a low-intensity[63] arm. The trial with the low-intensity intervention targeted younger teens (ages 12 to 15 years) and was the only trial reporting an STI outcome that included both sexually active and nonsexually active teens (males and females).[63] The moderate-intensity trial was limited to pregnant adolescents, most of whom were African American.[59] The remaining trials primarily included sexually active African American and/or Latina females, generally limited to ages 14 to 19 years. Two trials targeted adolescents with a recent STI at baseline, the highest risk category.[57,69] Because all sexually active adolescents are considered to be at increased risk, seven of the eight included comparisons targeted a group at increased risk.

STI incidence was reduced in all eight comparisons targeting adolescents (**Figure 4**), although results were not statistically significant in two trials.[59,63] We present detailed results in **Appendix C Table 3**. Pooled results showed a 62 percent reduction in the odds of acquiring an STI with high-intensity counseling after 12 months (OR, 0.38 [95% CI, 0.24 to 0.60]; I^2=65%; k=5) and a 43 percent reduction with the two moderate-intensity interventions (OR, 0.57 [95% CI, 0.37 to 0.86]; I^2=0%). Several trials reported only the relative difference in STI rate between groups (i.e., ORs and not STI rates in each group), and STI rates in the trials that did report them were highly variable. In trials with high-intensity interventions, reported STI rates at followup ranged from 13 to 40 percent in the control groups compared with 5 to 24 percent in the intervention groups.[63] Four of the trials were conducted in or recruited from primary care settings, and all reported reductions in the odds of acquiring an STI of 0.67 or less, although not all effects were statistically significant.[59,63,67,68]

The trial of pregnant adolescents and young adults found a statistically nonsignificant 33 percent reduction in the odds of acquiring an STI at the 12-month followup in adolescents.[59] The one trial that targeted younger adolescents (both sexually and presexually active youth) and reported STI rates found no statistically significant group differences in self-report of treatment for an STI, but overall event rates were very low (1.1% reporting STI treatment in the past 6 months in the intervention group vs. 5.8% in the control group at 9 months followup), resulting in limited statistical power.[63] This trial did find that a greater proportion of control group participants self-reported genital signs of possible STIs (6.8% in the control group vs. 0% in the intervention group).

Heterogeneity was high (I^2=65%; p=0.02) in the analysis of high-intensity interventions, primarily due to a very large effect in a fairly large good-quality trial by DiClemente and colleagues (OR, 0.17 [95% CI, 0.10 to 0.30]) (**Figure 4**).[68] Although the unadjusted rates of chlamydia in the study were similar between groups at the 12-month followup (2.1 per 100 person-months in the intervention group and 2.0 per 100 person-months in the control group), the baseline rates were higher in the intervention group. As such, the adjusted analysis shows a benefit of the intervention with a large effect. This study reported results separately for chlamydia (OR, 0.17 [95% CI, 0.03 to 0.92]), gonorrhea (OR, 0.14 [95% CI, 0.01 to 3.02]), and trichomoniasis (OR, 0.37 [95% CI, 0.09 to 1.46]), and did not report an overall STI incidence rate. We used results for the most prevalent STI (chlamydia) for our pooled analysis, which was the only effect that was statistically significant. Pooled results in sensitivity analyses using the results for gonorrhea and trichomoniasis instead of chlamydia were slightly attenuated, but they still showed a pooled 52 percent reduction in STIs for high-intensity interventions. Statistical heterogeneity was reduced to 0 percent when both the gonorrhea and trichomoniasis results were used.

The DiClemente trial involved four 4-hour group sessions developed specifically for African American adolescent girls. The intervention was delivered by a female African American health educator assisted by African American peer educators. The intervention covered knowledge and skills related to STI transmission and condom use, and included role playing of safe sex conversations, negotiating safer sex, and refusing unsafe sex. This intervention also covered the importance of healthy relationships. This intervention was compared with an intensity-matched general health intervention that received comparable favorability ratings (4.8 on a 5-point scale) as the sexual risk reduction counseling intervention, but was not as effective in reducing STIs.

Another trial, the Project RESPECT trial by Kamb and colleagues, tested both moderate- and high-intensity interventions in a high-risk setting (inner-city public STI clinic) and provided the only estimates for the effectiveness of behavioral counseling in mixed-gender sexually active adolescents.[58] Both interventions demonstrated sizeable reductions in STIs among the adolescent subgroup of both treatment arms and no differences between the moderate- and high-intensity arms; after 1 year, STI incidence was 17.2 percent in the high-intensity intervention group, 17.5 percent in the moderate-intensity intervention group, and 26.6 percent in the control group. This trial included HIV-negative adolescents and adults attending STI clinics in five different U.S. cities and agreeing to HIV testing. Just fewer than half of the participants were female, 59 percent were African American, and 19 percent were Latino. The moderate-intensity intervention included two 20-minute sessions and was based on the CDC recommendation for counseling in association with HIV testing. The high-intensity intervention added three additional individual 60-minute sessions tailored to each person's individual risks, developing and following up on specific risk reduction goals. This trial reported generally good methods and procedures, but suffered from low retention (e.g., 66% retention at the 1-year followup), which could cause under- or over-estimation of the true effect if those lost to followup had higher or lower than average risk for STIs.

Results in Adults

Nineteen trials (n=61,909) reported STI outcomes in adult populations (**Table 5; Appendix C Table 4**),[57-59,64,70-74,78-80,83-85,87-90] four of which had multiple treatment arms with different intensities.[58,71,79,84] Of the 23 comparisons, 10 examined high-intensity interventions,[57,58,64,71,73,79,84,85,88,89] seven examined moderate-intensity interventions,[58,59,70,71,80,87,90] and six examined low-intensity interventions.[72,74,78,79,83,84] We included all but three trials in the meta-analysis. Of the three we did not include, one only reported BV[74] (and was excluded because this outcome was substantially different from the other trials) and two trials did not provide sufficient data, reporting only that they found no statistically significant group differences.[70,84] Seven of the trials were conducted in or recruited from primary care.[59,70,72,79,83,85,89] The majority of the trials targeted patient populations at increased risk for STIs, but without requiring a recent STI diagnosis. Only two of the trials were in general primary care populations (one of which was included in the meta-analysis),[70,83] and five were limited to adults at highest risk based on a recent STI.[57,73,74,85,88] Several trials targeted narrow subpopulations, including one trial that targeted pregnant women,[59] two that targeted psychiatric patients,[64,82] one that targeted women with genital warts,[86] and one that targeted women who have sex with women and have BV.[74]

While only nine of the 23 comparisons were statistically significant, most showed an effect in the direction of a reduction in STIs in the intervention groups. The pooled effects for high-intensity interventions were statistically significant with relatively low statistical heterogeneity. High-intensity interventions resulted in a 30 percent reduction in the odds of acquiring an STI (OR, 0.70 [95% CI, 0.56 to 0.87]; k=9; I^2=23%) (**Figure 5**). The proportion of participants with an STI at followup in the high-intensity intervention groups ranged from 2 to 63 percent compared with 5 to 68 percent in the control groups. In a trial with an effect size close to the pooled effect,[57] 18 percent of control group participants contracted an STI over 12 months compared with 12 percent of intervention group participants. Three of these trials were conducted in primary care settings, with ORs ranging from 0.82 (95% CI, 0.46 to 1.45) to 0.48 (95% CI, 0.24 to 0.97).[79,85,89]

The pooled effects for low- and moderate-intensity trials did not show a reduction in the odds of acquiring an STI (**Figure 5**). Most of the low- and moderate-intensity trials did not reduce the odds of an STI, including three trials not included in the meta-analysis because of missing data. Two low- and two moderate-intensity interventions, however, did prove effective in preventing STIs.[78,79] For example, one large (n=40,282), good-quality randomized, controlled trial created a 23-minute video, "Safe in the City," that participants watched in the waiting room of STI clinics.[78] The video covered basic information on HIV/STI risk and prevention and attempted to build condom use skills, self-efficacy for condom use, and a positive attitude toward condom use. Vignettes with young couples of various race/ethnicity and sexual orientations demonstrated communication about partner notification and the acquisition, negotiation, and use of condoms. Control group participants attended the clinic when the video was not being shown. This trial found a small but statistically significant reduction in the proportion of participants with an STI. After an average of almost 15 months, 4.9 percent of intervention participants had an STI compared with 5.7 percent of control group participants (adjusted hazard ratio [HR], 0.91 [95% CI, 0.84 to 0.99]; unadjusted OR, 0.85 [95% CI, 0.73 to 0.99]), or a NNT of 123 (95% CI, 68 to 1,859). Planned subgroup analyses, however, revealed that the effect was statistically significant for men (adjusted HR, 0.88 [95% CI, 0.80 to 0.98]), but not for women (adjusted HR, 1.02 [95% CI, 0.86 to 1.21]).

Another trial by Jemmott and colleagues had five study arms, including an efficacious low-intensity intervention and a brief general health promotion arm as a control.[79] Two of the active intervention arms targeted skill building while two provided information without the opportunity to practice skills. One of the skill-based treatment arms was a high-intensity (≥3 hours), small-group session and the other was a 20-minute individual session. Similarly, the information-only intervention also had high- and low- intensity versions. Both of the high-intensity interventions included group brainstorming, videos, and interactive exercises. Both of the low-intensity interventions were tailored to the participant's individual risk factors. Using a priori contrasts, Jemmott and colleagues reported that STIs were lower in both of the skill-based intervention groups at 12 months (14% [high-intensity] and 15% [low-intensity]) than in the control group (27%). Furthermore, the two skill-based interventions were not statistically different from the two information-based interventions (19% [high-intensity] and 22% [low-intensity]).

Across the body of evidence, there was no clear relationship between the effect size and the number of sessions, reporting of condom negotiation or other communication as an intervention component, type of control group, or study quality, based on qualitative synthesis. More intensive approaches generally used group formats and brief interventions usually involved individual sessions. As such, we could not disentangle the effects of format from treatment intensity. Almost all trials relied on trained providers to deliver the intervention. These trials relied little on mailed or computer-based interventions, and the initial results in these media were not promising; a mail-only intervention[83] and a computer-based expert system[72] intervention both showed no benefit over the control group, with ORs of greater than 0.95 in both cases.

KQ 2. Do Behavioral Counseling Interventions to Prevent STIs Reduce Risky Sexual Behavior or Increase Protective Sexual Behavior?

Twenty-four trials reported an outcome related to condom use or unprotected sex (**Appendix C Tables 5** and **6**). Five trials were conducted in adolescents[57,63,66-68] and 19 were conducted in adults.[57-59,64,70-73,76,77,79,81-84,86-88,90] Additional behavioral outcomes, such as number of partners or initiation of sexual activity, were also reported in some studies (**Appendix C Tables 7** and **8**).[57,58,63-65,67,68,71,73,76,77,81,82,84-88,90] All behavioral outcomes were based on self-report.

Results in Adolescents

Six trials (n=3,030) reported sexual behavior outcomes. Three of these trials were high-intensity,[57,67,68] two were moderate-intensity,[65,66] and one was low-intensity.[63] Three of the five trials that reported effects on condom use or unprotected sex found a benefit of the intervention at followup (**Table 4**; **Appendix C Table 5**). Four of the five trials that reported other sexual behavior outcomes found group differences (**Table 4**; **Appendix C Table 7**).

All three of the high-intensity interventions reporting behavioral outcomes found beneficial effects on at least one behavioral outcome at some point of followup. These results, however, were not entirely consistent with a clear benefit.[57,67,68] For example, one trial found greater improvement with a skills-based group session than with the intensity-matched general health promotion control group on number of days of unprotected vaginal intercourse, number of sex partners, percentage with two or more partners in the past 3 months, and number of days of sex while under the influence of drugs or alcohol.[67] These groups differed, however, at only one of three followup assessments in all cases. Additionally, the other information-only intervention arm (an intensity- and content-matched informational group session) did not improve behavioral outcomes beyond the control condition. Intervention group participants in the trial with the most consistently positive results showed improvement on four of five sexual behavior outcomes: condom use at most recent intercourse, consistent condom use in the past 6 months, number of unprotected vaginal intercourse episodes, and proportion with new sex partners at both 6- and 12-month followup assessments.[68] This trial by DiClemente and colleagues (described under KQ 1) involved four 4-hour group sessions developed specifically for sexually active African American adolescent girls.

Only one[65] of the two moderate-intensity trials reporting sexual behavioral outcomes demonstrated a positive effect.[65,66] Young adolescents in the intervention group reported substantially reduced sexual activity at the 9-month followup (6.8% reporting any vaginal intercourse) compared with the control group (22%).[65] These results are based on self-report, however, which may represent an even greater risk for bias than usual, since mothers were involved in this intervention. This was a primary care–based intervention conducted in New York City clinics that primarily serve Latino populations. The intervention targeted mothers rather than the adolescents themselves and included one 30-minute session with an interventionist, two booster calls, and self-study modules addressing topics such as adolescent development and self-esteem, parenting strategies, communication and relationship-building between parent and teen, techniques to help adolescents cope with peer pressure, and adolescent sexual behavior. This study did not report outcomes related to condom use, unprotected sex, or STIs.

In contrast, the one low-intensity intervention trial conducted in adolescents (younger adolescents who were mostly not sexually active) reported that a higher proportion of intervention participants were sexually active at the 3-month followup (27% in the intervention group vs. 20% in the control group), but found no differences at the 9-month followup.[63] This trial also reported a higher proportion of participants using condoms at their most recent sexual intercourse in the intervention group (92%) than the control group (57%) at the 3-month followup, but not after 9 months.[63] This trial was conducted in five managed care pediatric clinics in the Washington, D.C., area for youth with scheduled general health examinations. Pediatricians participated in a 45-minute, one-on-one training session that covered the ASSESS (Awareness, Skills, Self-Efficacy/Self-esteem, Social support) model. Participants listened to a 15-minute, audiotaped risk assessment and education module before their visit, which was followed by a discussion with the pediatrician about sexual risk assessment, preventive counseling (with study materials to assist the pediatrician), and informational materials for teens.

Results in Adults

While the 21 trials (25 comparisons) in adults reporting behavioral outcomes were also mixed, the high-intensity interventions were fairly consistent in reporting beneficial results (**Table 5**). Our meta-analysis that included nine trials reporting condom use or related outcomes (11 comparisons) showed that the odds of condom use increased by 29 percent with high-intensity interventions (OR, 1.29 [95% CI, 1.13 to 1.48]; k=4; I^2=0%) (**Figure 6**), and the majority of the high-intensity interventions that were not included in the meta-analysis also showed group differences at one or more time points. The pooled effect was similar for moderate-intensity interventions (OR, 1.21 [95% CI, 1.00 to 1.46]; k=4; I^2=28%), but the two trials excluded from the meta-analysis had mixed findings. The pooled estimate for low-intensity trials was not statistically significant, and the trials that could not be included generally also showed no group differences. Effects in one study with multiple followup assessments were only statistically significant at 6 months (not 12 months), and several other trials reporting followup beyond 6 months showed no group differences.

When other sexual behavior outcomes were reported, results were almost always consistent with condom-related measures in the same study. The most commonly reported other sexual behavior outcome was number of sex partners. Other behavioral outcomes were usually improved with high-intensity interventions, and the results were mixed for moderate-intensity interventions. Other outcomes were sparsely reported in trials with low-intensity interventions.

KQs 1a, 2a. Are There Population or Intervention Characteristics That Influence the Effectiveness of Interventions?

Important Population Characteristics

Most of the included trials were conducted in fairly narrow populations, and some trials conducted subgroup analyses to examine whether the intervention was effective in particular subpopulations, which are described below. Only one trial performed interaction tests before delving into subgroup analyses.[59] As far as we could determine, only the Warner trial specifically described its subgroup analysis as being planned a priori and was adequately powered for the subgroup analysis.[78] In general, we found that some populations were poorly represented, but there was no clear evidence that interventions were less likely to be effective for any important subpopulation. Subgroup results were frequently consistent with overall study results.

Age

Trials and subgroup analyses targeting adolescents were highly likely to be effective, with fairly large effects. Most adolescent results showed reductions in odds of acquiring an STI close to 50 percent or greater. Of the three trials that covered a wide age range and reported separate effect estimates for adolescents and adults, all three found that the intervention was effective for adolescents but not adults in at least one treatment arm.[57-59] The pooled effects of counseling in adults for moderate- and high-intensity interventions demonstrated a reduction in STIs, but effect sizes tended to be smaller (generally <50%) and results were less consistently statistically significant than in adolescent trials or analyses.

The majority of the participants in the adult trials were young adults and the average age of participants was generally younger than 30 years. Several included trials were limited to young adults (ages 16 or 18 to 25 or 30 years). Pooled results for odds of acquiring an STI, however, were similar to those in adult trials with an average age of younger than 25 years (OR, 0.80 [95% CI, 0.60 to 1.08]; k=8; I^2=59%) (data not shown) or 25 years or older (OR, 0.78 [95% CI, 0.68 to 0.90]; k=8; I^2=22%) (data not shown). In contrast, the pooled OR for adolescents was 0.40 (95% CI, 0.26 to 0.60; k=7; I^2=56%) (data not shown). These analyses differ slightly from the intensity-stratified analyses reported under KQ 1 because they combined all levels of intervention intensity in one analysis and used only the single most intensive treatment arm for each trial within the age strata to get a single result for each age group, with no duplication of trials within age group. We found no data specific to older adults.

Sex

Many of the included trials were limited to females, which covers a wide range of intervention intensity and population risk groups. Three trials only included males, and all targeted different populations (mostly Caucasian males ages 15 to 18 years,[66] African American men ages 18 to 29 years with a newly diagnosed STI and a history of condom use,[87] and men ages 18 to 59 years with severe mental illness[82]), which limits generalizability. Several trials limited to women or girls showed a greater reduction in STIs in intervention versus control participants.[57,67-69,73,79,89] Female-only trials did not appear more or less likely to report statistically significant results than those in males or mixed-sex populations. In adolescents, however, only two trials included both boys and girls. The one trial that included only boys reported only behavioral outcomes. As such, there was insufficient data to assess differences in effects by gender in adolescents.[58,63]

Six adult trials reported results separately for males and females, and their findings were conflicting.[58,64,78,80,88,90] As described above, the Warner trial, which had planned a subgroup analysis a priori, found that the intervention reduced STIs in men (adjusted HR, 0.88 [95% CI, 0.80 to 0.98]), but not women (adjusted HR, 1.02 [95% CI, 0.86 to 1.21]).[78] Similarly, another trial found that the intervention benefited men on two behavioral outcomes at one of two followups, but not women for either outcome at either followup (3 or 5 months). This trial, however, found no group differences in the effect on STIs at either followup in either men or women.[88] In contrast, the third trial, which was conducted in persons with major mood or thought disorders, found that the intervention reduced unprotected vaginal intercourse in women, but not men. It found no differences between men and women, however, in two other behavioral outcomes or STIs.[64] Results did not differ between men and women in the final two trials that explored results by sex.[58,80]

Race/Ethnicity

Many of the included trials were limited to persons of African American and/or Latino descent because of the disease burden in these subpopulations. Most of the trials limited to only African Americans or Latinos were successful in reducing either STIs or risky sexual behaviors. We found no data specific to American Indians/Alaska Natives, despite the high prevalence of STIs in these populations.

Four adult trials reported exploratory subgroup analyses for different racial/ethnic groups, with inconsistent findings.[57-59,90] One of these trials that included two treatment arms found the high-intensity intervention was beneficial for white participants, but not participants with other racial/ethnic backgrounds. In contrast, the moderate-intensity intervention was beneficial for African Americans, but not those with other racial/ethnic backgrounds.[58] The other three trials were limited to or mostly African American or Latino women. A trial in pregnant women found no difference in treatment effectiveness between African American and Latino women,[59] but the third trial found slight differences in the pattern of results. While results were similar between African American and Mexican American women for unprotected vaginal intercourse, Mexican American women showed greater improvements in STI rates and African American women showed greater changes in monogamy and rapid partner turnover.[57] The final trial included both men and women and found no differences in effectiveness of the intervention by race. [90]

Sexual Orientation

Only two trials included a substantial proportion of MSM; however, they did not compare the effectiveness of the intervention between MSM and heterosexual men, although they did perform subgroup analyses and reported treatment effects separately.[78,90] Effect sizes were similar for MSM and heterosexual men in one trial;[78] however, the other reported a statistically significant deleterious effect in MSM (adjusted RR, 1.41 [98.3% CI, 1.05 to 1.90]) but no group differences in heterosexual men (adjusted RR, 0.81 [98.3% CI, 0.50 to 1.31).[90] This trial involved HIV testing as well as counseling, and was limited to participants with a negative HIV test. Thus, we cannot disentangle the effect of the HIV test from the counseling, but it may have been an important factor for MSM. Both trials involved brief, single-session interventions. One additional trial was limited to women who have sex with women and have BV, with the aim of reducing reinfection, but the intervention was no more effective in reducing subsequent BV infections than usual treatment plus information on adherence to Pap smear screening guidelines.[74]

Low-Income Urban Settings

Many trials were conducted in urban settings, and although indicators of socioeconomic status were not frequently reported, the trials that did report on these indicators generally reported low income and education levels. All of the trials in adolescents except one[66] were conducted in urban, mostly publicly-funded clinics. Adult trials were more varied; however, most trials with high-intensity interventions (which were generally effective) were also in low-income, urban populations.

Mental Illness and Depression

Two trials were limited to patients with mental illnesses and both provided high-intensity interventions.[64,82] Only one of these trials measured (self-reported) STIs in patients with a mood or thought disorder and substance use in the past year.[64] This trial did not find that the intervention reduced STIs. It did, however, report greater reductions in the number of acts of unprotected intercourse and the number of casual sex partners, but not total number of partners, compared with an intensity-matched substance use reduction intervention. This study conducted exploratory analyses showing that the reduction in unprotected intercourse was only among patients with a diagnosis of major depressive disorder, and not those with other diagnoses (mostly thought disorders). However, there were no differences in the effects on STIs or the two other behavioral outcomes between participants with depression and those with other diagnoses. The other trial was conducted in psychiatric patients with severe mental illnesses and found no reductions in risky sexual behaviors as a result of the intervention.[82]

Two additional trials performed exploratory subgroup analyses on participants who screened positive and negative for symptoms of depression at baseline; one trial included only adolescent girls and the other included adolescent and adult women.[57] Neither of the interventions in these trials directly addressed depression. Adolescent girls who screened positive for depressive symptoms showed improvements in multiple measures of condom use, which was consistent with the overall results of the trial.[68] In the subgroup with depressive symptoms in the mixed-aged trial, the intervention group had better outcomes than the control group for STI reinfection, mutual monogamy, and rapid partner turnover. There were, however, smaller or no group differences in these outcomes in women without depressive symptoms. The presence of depressive symptoms did not have an effect on the percentage of the intervention group reporting unsafe sex.[57]

History of Abuse

One trial was limited to adolescent girls with a history of abuse and a current STI, including 60 percent who had a history of sexual abuse.[69] The high-intensity intervention involved three one-on-one interviews with detailed assessment, two 3- to 4-hour group workshops based on ARRM, and three to five weekly support group meetings; a minimal treatment control group primarily covered treatment of STIs. Odds of acquiring an STI were reduced at 6- and 12-month followups; 4.8 percent of the intervention group had an STI between 6 and 12 months postbaseline compared with 13.2 percent of the control group. Exploratory subgroup analyses showed that the intervention effect was statistically significant for girls without a history of sexual abuse, but not for those with a history of sexual abuse.

Two additional high-intensity intervention trials conducted exploratory subgroup analyses of adolescent[68] or adult[81] women with history of gender-based or intimate partner violence. The trial in adolescents found that the intervention reduced the STI rate and improved condom use in multiple measures in girls with a history of gender-based violence, consistent with the overall study results.[68] Similarly, the trial in adult women found that the intervention was effective in reducing unprotected vaginal intercourse and an overall risk score in the short term (1 month) only, but not at 6- or 12-month followups in women with a history of intimate partner violence. This finding is consistent with the overall results of this trial.[81]

Important Intervention Characteristics

Intensity

Intensity influenced outcomes in included trials. High-intensity trials (contact time of >2 hours) were most likely to be effective. While moderate-intensity trials could also be effective, they were less consistently beneficial. Finally, low-intensity trials were least likely to be effective. A single session (which could be of low, moderate, or high intensity) in many cases was sufficient to reduce STIs.[67,78-80,87] In fact, pooled effect estimates were similar for trials with a single session (OR, 0.73 [95% CI, 0.57 to 0.94]; k=7; I^2=72%) (data not shown) and more than one session (OR, 0.62 [95% CI, 0.47 to 0.81]; k=13; I^2=69%) (data not shown).

Although most of the low-intensity trials did not show a benefit of treatment, there were two low-intensity trials that effectively reduced the odds of acquiring an STI—the large Warner trial of the video-based intervention, powered to detect a small effect,[78] and a low-intensity arm of a trial of African American women conducted by Jemmott and colleagues.[79] The latter trial included a 20-minute individualized and culturally tailored counseling session with trained African American nurse educators (who had received ≥8 hours of training in providing the intervention) compared with a general health promotion control.

Two other low-intensity trials provided similarly brief individualized sexual risk reduction counseling sessions, likely covering the same basic material as the Jemmott intervention, but did not show a benefit of treatment.[76,84] In one trial, Australian family physicians provided brief counseling to young adult patients of any risk level, guided by a study-provided checklist.[76] The length of the counseling session and the extent of the training provided to the physicians are unknown. In the other trial that included a single, brief one-on-one session, a trained nurse in an STI clinic conducted a 15-minute motivational interview targeted at increasing participants' condom use.[84] This was compared with a 15-minute informational session delivered primarily via DVD. Thus, there were some important differences between the Jemmott trial and the other two (ineffective) trials that may have contributed to the differences in effectiveness. The Jemmott trial, which was effective, provided the greatest degree of cultural tailoring, provided extensive training for the providers, and included a high-risk population. Thus, while only one of three low-intensity individualized brief interventions reduced STIs, there may be situations in which a single-session low-intensity intervention can be effective and for which replication is warranted.

Cultural Tailoring

Several trials reported cultural tailoring of their interventions.[57,67-69,73,75,79,85,87,89] While the majority of these trials were effective in reducing STIs, it is difficult to disentangle the effects of the cultural tailoring from other trial characteristics because these trials were generally also high-intensity interventions in high-risk patients. One good-quality trial conducted in adolescents had some of the most extensive cultural tailoring and some of the largest effects on both risky sexual behaviors and STI incidence. This study devoted the first of four 4-hour sessions to ethnic and gender pride.[68] The fact that the only low-intensity trial providing one-on-one counseling that was effective was a culturally tailored intervention is intriguing, but data were not available to isolate the effects of cultural tailoring. None of the included trials compared the culturally tailored intervention with a nontailored intervention.

Condom Negotiation or Communication

Most of the high-intensity and several of the moderate-intensity interventions included instruction in condom negotiation or communication. A subset of these provided practice role playing for condom negotiation or safe sex conversations,[57-59,67,71,73,75,79-82,84,85] and many also included hands-on practice correctly applying condoms with anatomical models.[57,58,67,71,73,79,82,84] Visual inspection of these trials compared with other trials showed no clear difference in effectiveness between those providing and not providing training in these areas. Meta-analysis limited to trials providing some type of condom negotiation or communication information (combining adolescent and adult studies, selecting only the highest-intensity intervention when there were multiple arms) resulted in a pooled OR of 0.60 (95% CI, 0.48 to 0.74; k=14; I^2=72%) (data not shown), while those that did not provide such training had a pooled OR of 0.71 (95% CI, 0.46 to 1.08; k=5; I^2=38%) (data not shown). CIs were highly overlapping between these two estimates, suggesting no clear differences in effectiveness between trials with and without condom negotiation and/or communication instruction. When we looked more narrowly at whether trials provided role playing of condom negotiation or safe sex conversations, CIs were again highly overlapping, suggesting no robust differences based on this single component (with role playing: OR, 0.68 [95% CI, 0.60 to 0.77]; k=9; I^2=0%; without role playing: OR, 0.55 [95% CI, 0.36 to 0.85]; k=10; I^2=80%) (data not shown). Two trials conducted by the same authors provided information but not opportunities to practice skills and had mixed results; one trial found larger effects in the interventions that provided skills practice, while the other did not.[67,79]

Relationship Issues

Three high-intensity intervention trials targeting nonwhite women addressed healthy relationships beyond safe sex communication.[57,69,81] These included a trial of African American adolescent girls with a history of abuse and an STI,[69] one targeting African American and Mexican American woman with an STI,[57] and one conducted in a Planned Parenthood clinic in a low-income, primarily nonwhite neighborhood in Brooklyn, New York.[81] These trials provided few details on how the topic was addressed, but described discussing what women want from a relationship and "avoiding partners who don't care."[57,81] All three trials were effective in reducing STI recurrence[57,69] or (when STIs were not reported) the number of occasions of unprotected intercourse.[81]

Counselor Characteristics

One trial examined the effect of counselor characteristics on the STI rate.[58] It found no association between STI rate and counselor characteristics (gender, ethnicity, education, counseling experience) or counselor-dyad characteristics (concordance of gender and ethnicity).[104] Counselors in this trial ranged in educational attainment from high school graduates to having a post-bachelor degree.

Setting

There were no apparent differences in effectiveness of trials conducted in primary care compared with other settings. Ten trials were conducted in primary care; there was a 43 percent reduction in the odds of acquiring an STI among the nine trials that could be included in the analysis (OR, 0.57 [95% CI, 0.38 to 0.86]; k=9; I^2=72%) (data not shown). In comparison, studies in other settings had a slightly smaller pooled effect, although the differences were not statistically significant (OR, 0.71 [95% CI, 0.58 to 0.87]; k=11; I^2=70%) (data not shown).

KQ 3. Are There Other Positive Outcomes Beside STI Incidence and Changes in Risky or Protective Sexual Behavior From Behavioral Counseling Interventions to Prevent STIs?

Nine fair- to good-quality trials (n=6,300) reported on other positive outcomes, including reducing unintended pregnancy,[59,63,68,70-72] reducing interpersonal violence,[81] increasing the use of oral contraceptives,[66,70,71] improving depressive symptoms,[75] and increasing testicular self-examinations (**Tables 4** and **5**; **Appendix C Tables 9** and **10**).[66] The interventions and populations varied across studies. We could not pool data because of the few studies and/or events.

Pregnancy was reported in six trials after 3 to 24 months of followup. Most were in low- or moderate-intensity trials that did not show reductions in STIs. Two studies were conducted in adolescents[63,68] and four were conducted in adults[70-72] or mixed ages.[59] Although fewer pregnancies were reported in the intervention group across all studies, only two studies showed a statistically significant difference between the intervention and control groups, at 6 months only.[59,68] One was a fair-quality study that delivered a moderate-intensity HIV prevention group intervention to pregnant women (ages 14 to 25 years) receiving prenatal care.[59] While this study reported fewer repeat pregnancies within 6 months postpartum in the intervention group than the two control groups (OR, 0.49 [95% CI, 0.27 to 0.91]), this difference was no longer statistically significant after 12 months postpartum. Furthermore, the intervention group differed from the usual care control group, but there was no difference between the intervention group and the attention-matched control group, which is the better test of the STI prevention component of the intervention. One good-quality study conducted in adolescents also showed a statistically significant difference in the number of pregnancies between groups at 6 months (OR, 0.38 [95% CI, 0.15 to 0.36]).[68] As in the study among pregnant women, however, the effects were no longer significant at 12 months.

Three trials targeted contraceptive use as well as STI prevention. Two of the trials conducted in young women found no differences in contraceptive use outcomes between intervention and control participants.[70,71] A fair-quality trial of a single moderate-intensity reproductive health consultation among adolescent males ages 15 to 18 years (n=1,195), however, found greater odds of using an effective form of birth control at the last intercourse in the intervention group than in the control group.[66] This intervention also increased the number of adolescents who performed a testicular self-examination triennially in the past year compared with the waitlist control group. The trial did not report outcomes of the testicular self-examination (e.g., identification of a mass, physician examination).

Only one good-quality study (Project FIO [The Future Is Ours]) examined the effects of two high-intensity gender-specific HIV/STI risk reduction interventions (four or eight sessions) on intimate partner violence among adult women (n=360).[81] At baseline, 42 percent of women had experienced intimate partner violence during the past 12 months.[105] These women were more likely to be older, of a minority or low socioeconomic status, and at higher risk for an STI (e.g., previous STI, lifetime use of drugs) than women who had never experienced abuse. There were no statistically significant differences in the number of women reporting abuse between the intervention and control groups at 6 and 12 months of followup. Thus, the interventions caused no further harms, but also did not provide a further benefit in regards to violence. There was also no difference between groups in the number of women who did or did not have a safer sex discussion with their partners and experienced subsequent physical abuse.

One fair-quality study among adult Chilean women (n=496) assessed depressive symptoms over the past week, as measured by the 20-item Center for Epidemiological Studies Depression Scale.[75] Participants in the high-intensity Mano a Mano-Mujer (Hand-to-Hand for Women) HIV-prevention intervention experienced significantly fewer depressive symptoms than the waitlist control group after 3 months of followup (p<0.05).

KQ 4. What Adverse Effects Are Associated With Behavioral Counseling Interventions to Prevent STIs in Primary Care?

Two fair-quality trials[84,85] and one good-quality trial[90] explicitly reported on adverse events (n=6,837). Two did not find any adverse events associated with the interventions; however, no further details were provided about the types of adverse effects examined or how they were ascertained.[84,85] The third trial reported more nonserious adverse events during the HIV test (e.g., syncope, pain) in the intervention group than in the control group (13 vs. 5 events).[90] The populations and interventions examined in these three trials were heterogeneous. One trial examined five combinations of brief and intensive motivational, informational, and behavioral workshops among adults (mean age, 29.2 years) who had engaged in risky sexual behavior during the past 3 months compared with a single information-only session.[84] Another trial examined the Well Women Program among low-income African American women (mean age, 38.1 years) with at least two previously diagnosed STIs in the past year.[85] The third trial examined a moderate-intensity HIV testing and risk reduction counseling intervention among 5,012 adults seeking services at an STI clinic.[90]

No study has shown an overall statistically significant paradoxical effect in the incidence of STIs or change in sexual or other behaviors. Only three trials found statistically nonsignificant increases in the odds of acquiring an STI.[59,88,90] Two of these three studies were relatively small and had fewer than 15 events in either arm.[59,88] However, as described above, a subgroup analysis in the largest of these trials showed a statistically significant deleterious effect on STI incidence in MSM, with 12.5 percent of control and 18.7 percent of intervention participants reporting an STI at followup (adjusted RR, 1.41 [98.3% CI, 1.05 to 1.90]).[90] Another trial that reported results separately for MSM and heterosexual men did not see a deleterious effect in MSM. There was no consistent evidence that the interventions increased sexual activity in adolescents; while one trial reported a short-term increase in the proportion of youth who were sexually active in the previous 3 months,[63] another reported a decrease (p<0.05),[65] and other trials found no differences in frequency or number of partners.[57,67,106] No trials reported on the time to sexual debut in younger adolescents.

CHAPTER 4. DISCUSSION

Summary of Evidence

This review included almost twice as many trials as the previous 2008 review because of the volume of data that has since been published, including considerably more data on the effectiveness of low- and moderate-intensity interventions, as well as additional trials including male participants. A summary of the evidence is shown in **Table 6**. Consistent with the previous review, we found that high-intensity (>2 hour) interventions were likely to reduce the rate of STIs in both adults and sexually active adolescents. Ten of the 16 high-intensity trials reported statistically significant reductions in the primary outcome (usually STIs). The odds of acquiring an STI were reduced by an estimated 30 percent in adults and by 62 percent in adolescents. Condom use also increased with high-intensity interventions, particularly in the short term (≤ 6 months). Several high-intensity trials that did not find reductions in STIs did find reductions in risky sexual behaviors. Effects on condom use were most consistently positive among adolescents receiving high-intensity interventions. Condom use and other behavioral outcomes, however, were all based on self-report, which may be biased because of social desirability effects.

While we included more than twice as many low- and moderate-intensity trials than in the previous review, most were still not efficacious. However, results from trials that did show a benefit were intriguing. Two trials that included high-intensity treatment counseling arms along with low- or moderate- intensity arms were successful in reducing STIs, and appeared to use the same interventionists for both treatment arms.[58,79] These interventionists may have had more extensive training and perhaps a deeper knowledge base than typical, which hints that highly skilled interventionists may be able to provide effective, less-intensive counseling. In addition, the positive effect of a 45-minute intervention targeting African American men is encouraging, given the relative lack of data for this subgroup in the previous review.[87] Also, the beneficial and highly disseminable low-intensity video intervention is promising for its potential reach.[78] These results warrant replication.

Single-session interventions could be efficacious, particularly those of moderate or high intensity. Pooled effects for single-session interventions (OR, 0.73 [95% CI, 0.57 to 0.94]) were similar to those with multiple sessions (OR, 0.62 [95% CI, 0.47 to 0.81]) and were consistent with results of another review of 20 single-session sexual risk reduction counseling interventions. Most of these studies were conducted in health care settings (OR, 0.65 [95% CI, 0.55 to 0.77]).[107]

We found no evidence suggesting that sexual risk reduction counseling is harmful for adults or adolescents. The two trials conducted in young adolescents (mostly before sexual debut) that reported the proportion of participants engaging in any sexual activity had contradictory results, and sparse reporting precludes us from drawing conclusions related to the concern that sexual risk reduction counseling in health care settings could increase sexual activity. A review of community-based, comprehensive, sexual risk reduction group interventions, however, found that these interventions reduced sexual activity (any: OR, 0.84 [95% CI, 0.75 to 0.95];

frequency: OR, 0.81 [95% CI, 0.72 to 0.90]).[108] We excluded most of these trials from our review because they were not conducted in health care settings, but the content of many of the interventions was quite similar to those in our review. Similarly, a meta-analysis of 174 trials that examined the effect of HIV risk reduction counseling on sexual activity concluded that sexual activity did not increase, and in fact decreased in some subgroups. However, these trials did not report adolescent results separately from adults.[109]

New data represented a wide range of population risk, and several studies included men, who were sparsely represented in the previous review. All but three of the included trials were conducted in the United States, most in primary care, STI clinics, or other reproductive health settings. While a few more trials included men, the majority still targeted young adult African American and Latina women. This is appropriate, considering the prevalence patterns of STIs in the United States. Interventions were frequently targeted to participants' gender and sociocultural background, although some mixed-gender trials (still primarily low-income and nonwhite) were also effective, such as the Project RESPECT trial and the brief video-based intervention in public STI clinic waiting rooms.[58,78]

Important Components of Sexual Risk Reduction Counseling

There is broad consensus that sexual risk reduction interventions should provide information on HIV/STI risk and prevention strategies, use techniques to enhance motivation and commitment to change, and help persons develop the skills necessary to reduce risky behaviors and engage in protective behaviors. These components are prominent in two widely cited models, ARRM and IMB.[110,111] Both of these theories are based on early examination of the AIDS risk reduction literature, and both have been tested in a number of trials. Almost all of the trials included in our review that used these models as the basis of their interventions were effective in reducing STIs or risky sexual behaviors.[57,64,69,73,81,87,88] More recent reviewers have supported the importance of these components and elucidated other characteristics believed to be important by researchers in the field. These are entirely consistent with both the ARRM and IMB models, such as a clear focus on sexual risk reduction, a theoretical model as the basis for the intervention development, sufficient magnitude and duration (exact magnitude and duration not specified), use of a variety of evidence-based intervention methods, information personalized to the participant, clear messages that strengthen values and norms that favor safety, tailoring to cultural and community norms, inclusion of the target group in program development, and clear goals and objectives.[112]

Unfortunately, we found little evidence to expressly confirm the importance of any of these components due to limited reporting of specific components in some cases. Likewise, clinical and methodological heterogeneity make it difficult to isolate the effects of any one characteristic or component. While two trials explored the effect of skills training rather than simply providing information, results from these trials were conflicting.[67,79] A review of the existing literature on sexual risk reduction counseling extracted information on moderator effects in 16 different reviews covering a wide range of target populations.[113] This review found that interventions tailored for target subgroups by sex, race/ethnicity, or sexual orientation frequently showed larger effect sizes than those addressing broader populations. Although the results were not entirely consistent across reviews, multiple meta-analyses found that matching facilitator race, skills training (e.g., condom use, safe sex negotiation, problem solving, goal setting), and the underlying theoretical model to all be associated with improved outcomes. A greater number of sessions was also reported as definitely or possibly being associated with better outcomes in several reviews.

Public Health Impact

The public health impact of sexual risk reduction counseling varies by community, based on such factors as the prevalence of STIs, the trend in prevalence over time, local norms regarding risky sexual behaviors, and the degree to which the target populations can be reached by an intervention. Nevertheless, estimated NNTs to prevent one STI infection are presented in **Table 7**, along with the estimated number of cases avoided per 1,000 persons receiving sexual risk reduction counseling. A high-intensity intervention in a setting with a baseline annual incidence rate of 15 percent could expect to need to treat 11 youths (95% CI, 9 to 18) over the course of 1 year to prevent one STI. In this scenario, an estimated 88 cases (95% CI, 55 to 110) per 1,000 adolescents would be prevented. Estimates are less precise for moderate-intensity interventions, however, since they are based on only two trials in adolescents. These estimates show a NNT of 17 (95% CI, 11 to 55) and 59 (95% CI, 19 to 89) cases prevented per 1,000 adolescents. These data for adolescents are based primarily on studies in African American and Latina girls. Between 2006 and 2010, there were 3.4 cases of chlamydia per 1,000 female adolescents. An estimated 75 to 85 percent of cases are asymptomatic in females, so reported cases may substantially underestimate the actual number of cases.[114] Therefore, assuming a national annual incidence of chlamydial infection of 5 percent among females ages 15 to 19 years, high-intensity counseling could prevent 31 cases per 1,000 female adolescents, or about 10,981 cases, in the United States. Thus, widespread adoption of high-intensity counseling in high-risk settings could prevent thousands of cases of chlamydia in adolescent girls, not to mention reductions in other STIs as well. While STI screening will largely prevent the long-term health sequelae of untreated STIs, young, low-income women tend to have difficulty accessing regular health care and are at risk for missing recommended STI screening. Therefore, widespread risk reduction counseling may also help prevent sequelae, such as PID and its associated pain and infertility, among some women with untreated STIs.

Twenty-five adults (95% CI, 17 to 59) would need high-intensity counseling to prevent one STI in a setting with an STI incidence of 15 percent. This would prevent 41 cases per 1,000 participants (95% CI, 61 to 17), again based largely on data from studies in nonwhite women. A study of 13 STI clinics in Los Angeles County seeing more than 32,000 unique patients in an 18-month period in 2006 to 2007 reported that 17 percent had an STI at their first visit.[115] Applying our estimate of 41 cases per 1,000 persons, approximately 1,300 STIs could potentially be prevented in this health care system, or a similarly sized system, with widespread adoption of high-intensity counseling.

The effects of primary care–based, sexual risk reduction counseling may also potentiate the effects of other types of community-level interventions. For example, the likelihood of benefit for condom distribution programs is enhanced with additional individual, small group, or community STI prevention interventions.[116] Given our finding that changes in condom use were primarily in the short-term only, STI prevention may be enhanced if persons hear risk-reduction messages from multiple sources, multiple times. Thus, even relatively modest effects may contribute to clinically important effects in communities where messages from other sources, such as community organizations and schools, are also frequently encountered.

The two low-intensity interventions that had a positive impact on STIs represent potentially important approaches that future studies should seek to replicate to confirm their effectiveness in populations at increased risk for STIs. One of these studies had a small absolute effect (14% reduction in STIs; 5.7% in the control group, 4.9% in the intervention group), but could fairly easily be widely implemented, potentially preventing thousands of the estimated 20 million new STIs cases annually.[2] However, dissemination efforts have not been as effective as hoped. The CDC Diffusion of Effective Behavioral Intervention project made substantial efforts to make this video freely available to STI clinics from the CDC Web site and inform STI clinics about its availability when trial results were published. Three to 5 months after publication, 76 of 212 identified STI clinics were surveyed to determine uptake. Twelve of the 76 clinics ordered the video and only five were actively using it at the time of the survey. Most clinics that had not ordered the video had not heard of it or its availability. The two barriers to using the video that were commonly reported by clinic managers were lack of equipment to show the video and shared waiting areas with other clinics or services (and therefore frequent presence of children).

The other low-intensity intervention included a culturally tailored, 20 minute, one-on-one skills-based counseling visit for sexually active African American women in a women's health clinic. This trial used female African American nurses who had extensive training in the delivery of the intervention. As such, while it likely does not have the potential to reach such a large audience as a waiting room video, it could substantially reduce STIs in targeted populations. While group-based interventions can have advantages such as peer support and staffing efficiency, individual visits are advantageous in that they do not require the patient to return for a separate visit and are likely easier to integrate into the clinical flow of a primary care clinic.

Acceptability of Sexual Risk Reduction Counseling

We identified limited data evaluating the acceptability of included interventions. While acceptability appeared to be good for participants, it was unclear for parents of adolescent participants. Eleven included trials reported on a measure related to acceptability,[58,63,66-68,70,75,76,83,84,86] and one longitudinal observational study assessed stigma in youth participating in a sexual risk reduction intervention.[117]

Two trials in sexually active adolescents compared satisfaction or favorability ratings between group-based general health information control conditions and sexual risk reduction counseling groups.[58,68] Both trials reported high favorability ratings in both intervention and control groups, with almost no differences between the groups. The only group difference noted was that one of these trials reported higher favorability ratings in the skills-based sexual risk reduction intervention (average rating, 4.67 on a 5-point scale) than either the information-based sexual risk reduction intervention (average rating, 4.46) or the general health control (average rating, 4.55).[58]

Two trials reported the rate at which parents refused to allow their children to participate in the study.[63,66] In one study of young adolescents (ages 12 to 15 years), 28 percent of parents reached by telephone to obtain study consent verbally refused or passively avoided consenting, although reasons for refusal were not reported.[63] In the other trial, conducted in adolescent males ages 15 to 18 years (not all sexually active), 8.6 percent of parents reached by telephone to obtain consent refused a reproductive health visit with a nurse educator.[66] Reasons for refusal were recorded for 47.8 percent of parents. Of those with a recorded reason for refusal, 64 percent said they were not interested, 28 percent said their child was too busy to participate, and a small number (not reported) explicitly objected to the sexual material covered in the study. Another study conducted in teens in the same health system during the same era reported a 16 percent refusal for a healthy lifestyle intervention of similar intensity, almost twice as high as the refusal rate for the reproductive health intervention. Recruitment in this latter study, however, took place face-to-face in the clinic as youth arrived for appointments rather than over the phone, which may have affected the refusal rate.[118] In summary, most parents did not object to the child's participation and we found no information on refusals related to the content of the intervention. Likewise, we found no suggestion that refusal rates were higher than expected for adolescent populations in health care settings.

The remaining trials reported some measure related to satisfaction or helpfulness in the intervention group only. All trials reported adequate to excellent acceptability.[58,70,75,76,83,84,86] For example, the Project RESPECT trial indicated that greater than 85 percent of participants surveyed about the interventions found that the sessions were "informative," "good," and "helpful."[58] Similarly, a study of a single counseling session and distribution of an educational leaflet for women with vulvoperineal warts reported that 95 percent of patients were satisfied or very satisfied with the leaflet compared with usual care.[86] In a trial of unintended pregnancy prevention and STI risk reduction among women at risk for unintended pregnancy, 82 percent indicated it was helpful to talk about contraception, 90 percent felt that the health educator focused on their individual concerns, and 93 percent felt that the health educator addressed all of their questions.[70]

One study reported participants' ease of talking to a doctor about sex and preferred source of information about sex and related problems.[76] This study of a brief individual session with a primary care provider indicated that the majority of participants found it to be "very easy" (22%) or "somewhat easy" (48%) to talk to their doctor about sex. Eleven percent of participants reported that it was "difficult" or "very difficult" to discuss sex with their doctor. Intervention group participants indicated they preferred information about sex from their usual primary care provider (49%), followed by sexual health clinic (12%) and family planning clinic (12%).

A longitudinal study not included in this review reported on the relationship between HIV-related stigma and gains in HIV knowledge in teens participating in a multilevel, multisite HIV risk reduction intervention.[117] The intervention was not designed to reduce HIV-related stigma, but rather to compare the intervention's effect on HIV stigma with that of the health promotion control. Intervention participants showed more reduction in stigma compared with control participants (p<0.05). Additionally, researchers found that higher baseline HIV-related stigma was related to smaller gains in HIV knowledge, suggesting that stigma in teens regarding HIV may affect their ability to internalize information regarding HIV. This study suggests that participation in a HIV risk reduction intervention is more likely to reduce stigma than increase it, although data are extremely limited.

Limitations of the Review

Limitations of Our Report

One important limitation of the data on behavioral outcomes was that they were based on self-report. Indeed, a study of adolescent and young adult women who self-reported using condoms 100 percent of the time found a biomarker for unprotected vaginal intercourse within 14 days on swabs collected from 34 percent of participants.[119] Sexual behavior outcomes may be especially vulnerable to biases related to social desirability, given the personal nature of sexual behavior and the risk for feeling shame or stigma as a result of particular behaviors. This is likely compounded for adolescents, many of whom may wish to keep their sexual activity hidden from their parents and other adults. While parental involvement in interventions targeting young adolescents remains an area of potential value for further exploration, strenuous efforts to ensure confidentiality may still fail to win confidence from participants and lead to biased findings.

Another limitation of our review is that we excluded comparative effectiveness trials, including some that barely exceeded our minimum threshold for a control group. We excluded 41 publications because of comparative effectiveness (**Appendix B**), one of the most common reasons for exclusion among studies that made it through the title and abstract screening process. Some of these studies may have been excluded for other reasons as well. Several trials that were excluded for comparative effectiveness tested different formats (e.g., group vs. individual, interactive computer vs. printed materials) for providing the same content and rarely found group differences. Trials that reported more and less intensive interventions, however, frequently reported greater reductions in risky sexual behaviors or STIs with more intensive interventions. Few trials attempted to isolate the effects of a single component of the intervention.

Limitations of the Data on Populations

Some populations were not well represented in the included trials, even though they were at high risk for acquiring STIs. One notable population that was minimally represented in these studies, and missing entirely from high-intensity trials, was MSM. We excluded all trials that targeted MSM, most because they were not conducted in health care settings. However, there is a substantial body of literature on HIV/STI prevention in MSM in community settings. The Community Preventive Services Task Force found that community-based individual-, group-, and community-level interventions were effective in reducing risk for STIs in MSM.[120] Of the few health care–based trials in MSM we identified, most were excluded because the control group exceeded our a priori threshold for intervention intensity (≤15 minutes). The trial that came closest to meeting our inclusion criteria was conducted in a health clinic that used a 20-minute control condition.[121] In this trial, MSM with STIs were randomized to a single, one-on-one 20-minute session consistent with CDC guidelines or to both the 20-minute visit and a 1-day HIV prevention workshop. The intervention did not reduce the risk for subsequent infections over the course of the following year. In fact, there was a greater proportion of STIs in the intervention group (31%) than the control group (21%), although this difference was only marginally statistically significant (adjusted OR, 1.66 [95% CI, 1.00 to 2.74]). There are numerous studies in MSM currently underway (**Appendix D**), including one large (n=4,000) technology-based intervention that may meet inclusion criteria for future USPSTF reviews.

Illicit drug users and adults with psychiatric conditions are other high-risk populations that were not well represented in our review. We included only two trials in psychiatric patients, one of which was further limited to illicit drug users with mental illness.[64,82] Most trials in adults with mental illness focused on populations recruited from residential or institutional settings and, as such, did not meet inclusion criteria. Similarly, trials targeting illicit drug users were generally conducted in community or inpatient settings or were excluded because their control condition was too intensive (e.g., two brief, individually tailored sessions using CDC guidelines for HIV counseling and testing, with an estimated contact time of >15 minutes). Meta-analyses of HIV prevention interventions in illicit drug users indicate modest benefit of risk reduction counseling in this population.[122,123] While most trials included in the meta-analysis were not conducted in health care settings, it did identify 12 trials in drug treatment or other health care settings. However, it did not report results separately for these studies.[122]

We also found no primary care–relevant evidence for American Indians/Alaska Natives or adults age 50 years and older. Rates of chlamydia and gonorrhea in American Indians/Alaska Natives are second only to African Americans nationwide, and rates of both of these infections in Alaska are among the highest in the United States. Nevertheless, we identified no health care–based efforts that included substantial numbers of American Indians or Alaska Natives. While older adults do not represent a population with high absolute rates of STIs, the increase in STI rates in recent years suggests that interventions targeting this age group may be needed.[34]

Limitations of the Data on Other STI Prevention Strategies

In addition to not covering all important subpopulations because of limitations of the literature, we also did not cover a number of important STI risk reduction strategies that cannot be implemented in health care settings or go beyond risk reduction counseling. For example, programs to encourage STI and HIV testing and partner notification programs aim to reduce STIs by increasing awareness and treatment of STIs that are frequently asymptomatic.

Similarly, the Community Preventive Services Task Force recommends partner notification by provider referral for persons with HIV (available at www.thecommunityguide.org). We did not include interventions to increase safe sex behaviors in persons with HIV because of limited applicability to most primary care settings. If effective, such programs may not only reduce the spread of HIV to HIV-negative persons, but may also reduce the rate of other STIs in the HIV-positive population. This may be especially important since HIV-positive persons are highly susceptible to STIs.[8] Condom distribution programs can also be effective for reducing STI rates, but were not included in this review.[116]

We also did not cover school-based interventions. A review of school-based sexual risk reduction interventions in adolescents did not demonstrate a beneficial effect on self-reported sexual behaviors, although knowledge generally increased. Reviewers noted that interventions were frequently not implemented as intended due to variability in school culture, support from school administration, and enthusiasm and skill of teachers and other interventionists.[124]

The CDC maintains a regularly updated compendium of evidence-based individual-, group-, and community-level interventions and associated dissemination materials, targeting a wide range of risk populations and risk reduction strategies.[125] This is an excellent source for interventions that have been empirically tested, and includes many interventions conducted in community-based settings that were not included in our review.

Future Research Needs

While the body of literature on primary care–relevant sexual risk reduction counseling is relatively mature, there are still some important evidence gaps and promising single-study findings that need replication. Most evidence comes from adolescents and other high-risk populations, particularly high-risk women. While interventions tailored to fairly narrow populations tend to show larger effects than those designed for wider administration, broadly targeted interventions have the potential for greater reach and should not be abandoned. Thus, more data are needed in mixed-gender and other broad-based interventions that could be implemented in or linked to primary care.

We found minimal data on interventions conducted in health care settings targeted toward primary prevention in younger adolescents. This is another area that has the potential for broad reach, but trials would require large samples and long-term followup to observe initiation of sexual activity and exposure to STIs sufficient to demonstrate a public health impact. In particular, replicating the promising intervention that targeted mothers of younger adolescents with longer followup would be useful, so that risky sexual behavior outcomes and STI rates could be assessed.

While high-intensity interventions were most likely to be efficacious, there were two low-intensity interventions that reduced STIs. Replicating these two trials should be a priority.[78,79] One trial was a 20-minute culturally tailored intervention that employed highly trained facilitators.[79] This trial demonstrated a beneficial effect in African American women. The other intervention involved a video that is freely available from the CDC. While some clinics may prefer not to show such a video to everyone in their waiting area, this intervention may be amenable to adaptation for personal mobile devices, whether in a waiting room, examination room, or at home. Other uses of interactive mobile, Web-based, or other automated expert systems have been only minimally assessed in the health care context and represent potentially fruitful avenues for exploration. An example of one such intervention is a 12-episode soap opera streamed to smartphones of young urban African American women.[126] This trial, which recruited from an STI clinic and four other nonhealth care–based community settings, found that participants recruited from the STI clinic showed greater reductions in risky sexual behaviors than those recruited from other community sources, suggesting that such interventions in a health care context may be promising.

Conclusion

Moderate- and high-intensity interventions in primary care or similar health care settings can reduce STIs and risky sexual behaviors, particularly in sexually active adolescents and high-risk adults. While low-intensity interventions generally do not reduce STI risk, some approaches show promise and trial replication should be pursued. Data on primary prevention in presexually active adolescents are sparse. We found no evidence that sexual risk reduction counseling is harmful. These findings are consistent with the results of the previous USPSTF review on this topic. This review expands upon that review's findings with the addition of almost twice as many included trials, many with both low- and moderate-intensity interventions.

REFERENCES

1. Centers for Disease Control and Prevention. Sexually transmitted diseases treatment guidelines, 2010. *MMWR Recomm Rep.*. 2010;59(RR-12):1-110.
2. Centers for Disease Control and Prevention. Incidence, Prevalence, and Cost of Sexually Transmitted Infections in the United States. Atlanta, GA: Centers for Disease Control and Prevention; 2013.
3. Forhan SE, Gottlieb SL, Sternberg MR, et al. Prevalence of sexually transmitted infections among female adolescents aged 14 to 19 in the United States. *Pediatrics.* 2009;124(6):1505-12. PMID: 19933728.
4. Chesson HW, Gift TL, Owusu-Edusei K Jr, et al. A brief review of the estimated economic burden of sexually transmitted diseases in the United States: inflation-adjusted updates of previously published cost studies. *Sex Transm Dis.* 2011;38(10):889-91. PMID: 21934557.
5. Centers for Disease Control and Prevention. Sexually Transmitted Disease Surveillance 2011. Atlanta, GA: U.S. Department of Health and Human Services; 2012.
6. Centers for Disease Control and Prevention. HIV in the United States: At a Glance. Atlanta, GA: Centers for Disease Control and Prevention; 2012.
7. Centers for Disease Control and Prevention. HIV Surveillance Report, 2009. Atlanta, GA: Centers for Disease Control and Prevention; 2011.
8. Centers for Disease Control and Prevention. The Role of STD Prevention and Treatment of HIV Prevention. Atlanta, GA: Centers for Disease Control and Prevention; 2010.
9. Centers for Disease Control and Prevention. HIV Prevention in the United States. Atlanta, GA: Centers for Disease Control and Prevention; 2009.
10. Centers for Disease Control and Prevention. Genital Herpes: CDC Fact Sheet. Atlanta, GA: Centers for Disease Control and Prevention; 2013.
11. Office of Population Affairs. Genital Herpes Fact Sheet. Washington, DC: U.S. Department of Health and Human Services; 2012.
12. Centers for Disease Control and Prevention. Disease Burden From Viral Hepatitis A, B, and C in the United States. Atlanta, GA: Centers for Disease Control and Prevention; 2009.
13. Centers for Disease Control and Prevention. Viral Hepatitis Surveillance: United States, 2010. Atlanta, GA: Centers for Disease Control and Prevention; 2012.
14. Centers for Disease Control and Prevention. Trichomoniasis: CDC Fact Sheet. Atlanta, GA: Centers for Disease Control and Prevention; 2012.
15. Chandra A, Martinez GM, Mosher WD, et al. Fertility, family planning, and reproductive health of U.S. women: data from the 2002 National Survey of Family Growth. *Vital Health Stat.* 2005; 23(25):1-160. PMID: 16532609.
16. Martinez GM, Chandra A, Abma JC, et al. Fertility, contraception, and fatherhood: data on men and women from cycle 6 (2002) of the 2002 National Survey of Family Growth. *Vital Health Stat.* 2006; 23(26):1-142. PMID: 16900800.
17. Copen CE, Chandra A, Martinez G. Prevalence and timing of oral sex with opposite-sex partners among female and males aged 15-24 years: United States, 2007-2010. *Natl Health Stat Rep.* 2012(56):1-14.

18.   Kaestle CE, Halpern CT, Miller WC, et al. Young age at first sexual intercourse and sexually transmitted infections in adolescents and young adults. *Am J Epidemiol.* 2005;161(8):774-80. PMID: 15800270.

19.   Tu W, Batteiger BE, Wiehe S, et al. Time from first intercourse to first sexually transmitted infection diagnosis among adolescent women. *Arch Pediatr Adolesc Med.* 2009;163(12):1106-11. PMID: 19996047.

20.   World Health Organization. Sexually Transmitted Infections. Geneva, Switzerland: World Health Organization; 2011.

21.   Fung M, Scott KC, Kent CK, et al. Chlamydial and gonococcal reinfection among men: a systematic review of data to evaluate the need for retesting. *Sex Transm Infect.* 2007;83(4):304-9. PMID: 17166889.

22.   Hosenfeld CB, Workowski KA, Berman S, et al. Repeat infection with chlamydia and gonorrhea among females: a systematic review of the literature. *Sex Transm Dis.* 2009;36(8):478-89. PMID: 19617871.

23.   Centers for Disease Control and Prevention. Sexually Transmitted Disease Surveillance 2010. Atlanta, GA: Centers for Disease Control and Prevention; 2011.

24.   Centers for Disease Control and Prevention. Vital signs: HIV infection, testing, and risk behaviors among youths--United States. *MMWR Morb Mortal Wkly Rep.* 2012;61(47):971-6. PMID: 23190571.

25.   Centers for Disease Control and Prevention. STDs in Men Who Have Sex With Men. Atlanta, GA: Centers for Disease Control and Prevention; 2011.

26.   Chesson HW, Kent CK, Owusu-Edusei K Jr, et al. Disparities in sexually transmitted disease rates across the "eight Americas." *Sex Transm Dis.* 2012;39(6):458-64. PMID: 22592831.

27.   Korzeniewski K. Sexually transmitted infections among army personnel in the military environment. In: Malla N (ed). Sexually Transmitted Infections. Croatia: InTech; 2012. p. 165-82.

28.   Carey MP, Weinhardt LS, Carey KB. Prevalence of infection with HIV among the seriously mentally ill: review of research and implications for practice. *Prof Psychol Res Pract.* 1995;26:262-8.

29.   Hammett TM, Kennedy S, Kuck S. National Survey of Infectious Disease in Correctional Facilities: HIV and Sexually Transmitted Diseases. Washington, DC: U.S. Department of Justice; 2007.

30.   Beltrami J, Wright-DeAguero L, Fullilove M, et al. Substance Abuse and the Spread of Sexually Transmitted Diseases. Washington, DC: Institute of Medicine Committee on Prevention and Control for Sexually Transmitted Diseases; 2012.

31.   Homma Y, Wang N, Saewyc E, et al. The relationship between sexual abuse and risky sexual behavior among adolescent boys: a meta-analysis. *J Adolesc Health.* 2012;51(1):18-24. PMID: 22727072.

32.   Bobashev GV, Zule WA, Osilla KC, et al. Transactional sex among men and women in the south at high risk for HIV and other STIs. *J Urban Health.* 2009;86(Suppl 1):32-47. PMID: 19513853.

33.   Jones DL, Irwin KL, Inciardi J, et al. The high-risk sexual practices of crack-smoking sex workers recruited from the streets of three American cities. The Multicenter Crack Cocaine and HIV Infection Study Team. *Sex Transm Dis.* 1998;25(4):187-93. PMID: 9564720.

34.   Minichiello V, Rahman S, Hawkes G, et al. STI epidemiology in the global older population: emerging challenges. *Perspect Public Health.* 2012;132(4):178-81. PMID: 22729008.

35.   Centers for Disease Control and Prevention. HIV/AIDS Among Persons Aged 50 and Older. Atlanta, GA: Centers for Disease Control and Prevention; 2008.

36.   Jameson M. Seniors' sex lives are up--and so are STD cases. Orlando, FL: Orlando Sentinal; 2011.

37.   Wimberly YH, Hogben M, Moore-Ruffin J, et al. Sexual history-taking among primary care physicians. *J Natl Med Assoc.* 2006;98(12):1924-9. PMID: 17225835.

38.   Effective Interventions: HIV Prevention That Works. Silver Spring, MD: Effective Interventions; 2013. Accessed at http://www.effectiveinterventions.org/en/Home.aspx on 15 September 2014.

39.   Miller KS, Wyckoff SC, Lin CY, et al. Pediatricians' role and practices regarding provision of guidance about sexual risk reduction to parents. *J Prim Prev.* 2008;29(3):279-91. PMID: 18461458.

40.   Millstein SG, Igra V, Gans J. Delivery of STD/HIV preventive services to adolescents by primary care physicians. *J Adolesc Health.* 1996;19(4):249-57. PMID: 8897102.

41.   Ashton MR, Cook RL, Wiesenfeld HC, et al. Primary care physician attitudes regarding sexually transmitted diseases. *Sex Transm Dis.* 2002;29(4):246-51. PMID: 11912468.

42.   Hansen L, Barnett J, Wong T, et al. STD and HIV counseling practices of British Columbia primary care physicians. *AIDS Patient Care STDS.* 2005;19(1):40-8. PMID: 15665634.

43.   Mark H, Irwin K, Sternberg M, et al. Providers' perceived barriers to sexually transmitted disease care in 2 large health maintenance organizations. *Sex Transm Dis.* 2008;35(2):184-9. PMID: 18046264.

44.   Bull SS, Rietmeijer C, Fortenberry JD, et al. Practice patterns for the elicitation of sexual history, education, and counseling among providers of STD services: results from the Gonorrhea Community Action Project (GCAP). *Sex Transm Dis.* 1999;26(10):584-9. PMID: 10560723.

45.   Langille DB, Mann KV, Gailiunas PN. Primary care physicians' perceptions of adolescent pregnancy and STD prevention practices in a Nova Scotia county. *Am J Prev Med.* 1997;13(4):324-30. PMID: 9236972.

46.   Chung PJ, Lee TC, Morrison JL, et al. Preventive care for children in the United States: quality and barriers. *Annu Rev Public Health.* 2006;27:491-515. PMID: 16533127.

47.   Kurth AE, Holmes KK, Hawkins R, et al. A national survey of clinic sexual histories for sexually transmitted infection and HIV screening. *Sex Transm Dis.* 2005;32(6):370-6. PMID: 15912084.

48.   Office of the Surgeon General. The Surgeon General's Call to Action to Promote Sexual Health and Responsible Sexual Behavior. Rockville, MD: Office of the Surgeon General, Office of Population Affairs; 2001. PMID: 20669514.

49.   Division of STD Prevention. Division of STD Prevention Strategic Plan, 2008-2013. Atlanta, GA: Centers for Disease Control and Prevention; 2008.

50.   Centers for Disease Control and Prevention. Sexually Transmitted Diseases (STDs): Projects and Initiatives. Atlanta, GA: Centers for Disease Control and Prevention; 2010.

51. U.S. Department of Health and Human Services. Healthy People 2020 Summary of Objectives: Sexually Transmitted Diseases. Washington, DC: U.S. Department of Health and Human Services; 2012.

52. Meyers D, Wolff T, Gregory K, et al. USPSTF recommendations for STI screening. *Am Fam Physician.* 2008;77(6):819-24. PMID: 18386598.

53. U.S. Preventive Services Task Force. Behavioral counseling to prevent sexually transmitted infections: U.S. Preventive Services Task Force recommendation statement. *Ann Intern Med.* 2008;149(7):491-6. PMID: 18838729.

54. Lin JS, Whitlock E, O'Connor E, et al. Behavioral counseling to prevent sexually transmitted infections: a systematic review for the U.S. Preventive Services Task Force. *Ann Intern Med.* 2008;149(7):497-9. PMID: 18838730.

55. World Health Organization. International Human Development Indicators. Geneva: World Health Organization; 2013. Accessed at http://hdr.undp.org/en/data on 15 September 2014.

56. Harris RP, Helfand M, Woolf SH, et al. Current methods of the U.S. Preventive Services Task Force: a review of the process. *Am J Prev Med.* 2001;20(3 Suppl):21-35. PMID: 11306229.

57. Shain RN, Piper JM, Newton ER, et al. Even if you build it, we may not come: correlates of non-attendance at a sexual risk reduction workshop for STD clinic patients. *N Engl J Med.* 1999;340(2):93-100. PMID: 9887160.

58. Kamb ML, Fishbein M, Douglas JM Jr, et al. Efficacy of risk-reduction counseling to prevent human immunodeficiency virus and sexually transmitted diseases: a randomized controlled trial. Project RESPECT Study Group. *JAMA.* 1998;280(13):1161-7. PMID: 9777816.

59. Kershaw TS, Magriples U, Westdahl C, et al. Pregnancy as a window of opportunity for HIV prevention: effects of an HIV intervention delivered within prenatal care. *Am J Public Health.* 2009;99(11):2079-86. PMID: 19762662.

60. Higgins JP, Thompson SG. Quantifying heterogeneity in a meta-analysis. *Stat Med.* 2002;21(11):1539-58. PMID: 12111919.

61. Higgins JP, Green S (eds). Cochrane Handbook for Systematic Reviews of Interventions. West Sussex, England: Cochrane Collaboration; 2012.

62. Borenstein M, Hedges LV, Higgins JP, Rothstein HR. Introduction to Meta-Analysis. West Sussex, England: Wiley & Sons; 2009.

63. Boekeloo BO, Schamus LA, Simmens SJ, et al. A STD/HIV prevention trial among adolescents in managed care. *Pediatrics.* 1999;103(1):107-15. PMID: 9917447.

64. Carey MP, Carey KB, Maisto SA, et al. Reducing HIV-risk behavior among adults receiving outpatient psychiatric treatment: results from a randomized controlled trial. *J Consult Clin Psychol.* 2004;72(2):252-68. PMID: 15065959.

65. Guilamo-Ramos V, Bouris A, Jaccard J, et al. A parent-based intervention to reduce sexual risk behavior in early adolescence: building alliances between physicians, social workers, and parents. *J Adolesc Health.* 2011;48(2):159-63. PMID: 21257114.

66. Danielson R, Marcy S, Plunkett A, et al. Reproductive health counseling for young men: what does it do? *Fam Plann Perspect.* 1990;22(3):115-21. PMID: 2379568.

67. Jemmott JB III, Jemmott LS, Braverman PK, et al. HIV/STD risk reduction interventions for African American and Latino adolescent girls at an adolescent medicine clinic: a randomized controlled trial. *Arch Pediatr Adolesc Med.* 2005;159(5):440-9. PMID: 15867118.

68. DiClemente RJ, Wingood GM, Harrington KF, et al. Efficacy of an HIV prevention intervention for African American adolescent girls: a randomized controlled trial. *JAMA.* 2004;292(2):171-9. PMID: 15249566.

69. Champion JD, Collins JL. Comparison of a theory-based (AIDS Risk Reduction Model) cognitive behavioral intervention versus enhanced counseling for abused ethnic minority adolescent women on infection with sexually transmitted infection: results of a randomized controlled trial. *Int J Nurs Stud.* 2012;49(2):138-50. PMID: 21937041.

70. Petersen R, Albright J, Garrett JM, et al. Pregnancy and STD prevention counseling using an adaptation of motivational interviewing: a randomized controlled trial. *Perspect Sex Reprod Health.* 2007;39(1):21-8. PMID: 17335378.

71. Berenson AB, Rahman M. A randomized controlled study of two educational interventions on adherence with oral contraceptives and condoms. *Contraception.* 2012;86(6):716-24. PMID: 22840278.

72. Peipert JF, Redding CA, Blume JD, et al. Tailored intervention to increase dual-contraceptive method use: a randomized trial to reduce unintended pregnancies and sexually transmitted infections. *Am J Obstet Gynecol.* 2008;198(6):630-8. PMID: 18395692.

73. Shain RN, Piper JM, Holden AE, et al. Prevention of gonorrhea and chlamydia through behavioral intervention: results of a two-year controlled randomized trial in minority women. *Sex Transm Dis.* 2004;31(7):401-8. PMID: 15215694.

74. Marrazzo JM, Thomas KK, Ringwood K. A behavioural intervention to reduce persistence of bacterial vaginosis among women who report sex with women: results of a randomised trial. *Sex Transm Infect.* 2011;87(5):399-405. PMID: 21653935.

75. Cianelli R, Ferrer L, Norr KF, et al. Mano a Mano-Mujer: an effective HIV prevention intervention for Chilean women. *Health Care Women Int.* 2012;33(4):321-41. PMID: 22420675.

76. Proude EM, D'Este C, Ward JE. Randomized trial in family practice of a brief intervention to reduce STI risk in young adults. *Fam Pract.* 2004;21(5):537-44. PMID: 15367476.

77. Wenger NS, Greenberg JM, Hilborne LH, et al. Effect of HIV antibody testing and AIDS education on communication about HIV risk and sexual behavior. A randomized, controlled trial in college students. *Ann Intern Med.* 1992;117(11):905-11. PMID: 1443951.

78. Warner L, Klausner JD, Rietmeijer CA, et al. Effect of a brief video intervention on incident infection among patients attending sexually transmitted disease clinics. *PLoS Med.* 2008;5(6):e135. PMID: 18578564.

79. Jemmott LS, Jemmott JB, III, O'Leary A. Effects on sexual risk behavior and STD rate of brief HIV/STD prevention interventions for African American women in primary care settings. *Am J Public Health.* 2007;97(6):1034-40. PMID: 17463391.

80. Neumann MS, O'Donnell L, Doval AS, et al. Effectiveness of the VOICES/VOCES sexually transmitted disease/human immunodeficiency virus prevention intervention when administered by health department staff: does it work in the "real world"? *Sex Transm Dis.* 2011;38(2):133-9. PMID: 20729794.

81. Ehrhardt AA, Exner TM, Hoffman S, et al. A gender-specific HIV/STD risk reduction intervention for women in a health care setting: short- and long-term results of a randomized clinical trial. *AIDS Care.* 2002;14(2):147-61. PMID: 11940275.

82. Berkman A, Pilowsky DJ, Zybert PA, et al. HIV prevention with severely mentally ill men: a randomised controlled trial. *AIDS Care.* 2007;19(5):579-88. PMID: 17505917.

83. Scholes D, McBride CM, Grothaus L, et al. A tailored minimal self-help intervention to promote condom use in young women: results from a randomized trial. *AIDS.* 2003;17(10):1547-56. PMID: 12824793.

84. Carey MP, Senn TE, Vanable PA, et al. Brief and intensive behavioral interventions to promote sexual risk reduction among STD clinic patients: results from a randomized controlled trial. *AIDS Behav.* 2010;14(3):504-17. PMID: 19590947.

85. Marion LN, Finnegan L, Campbell RT, et al. The Well Woman Program: a community-based randomized trial to prevent sexually transmitted infections in low-income African American women. *Res Nurs Health.* 2009;32(3):274-85. PMID: 19373824.

86. Cortes-Bordoy J, Vidart JA, Coll-Capdevila C, et al. Usefulness of an educational leaflet to modify sexual risk behaviour in women with external genital warts. *Eur J Dermatol.* 2010;20(3):339-44. PMID: 20146965.

87. Crosby R, DiClemente RJ, Charnigo R, et al. A brief, clinic-based, safer sex intervention for heterosexual African American men newly diagnosed with an STD: a randomized controlled trial. *Am J Public Health.* 2009;99(Suppl 1):S96-103. PMID: 19218185.

88. Boyer CB, Barrett DC, Peterman TA, et al. Sexually transmitted disease (STD) and HIV risk in heterosexual adults attending a public STD clinic: evaluation of a randomized controlled behavioral risk-reduction intervention trial. *AIDS.* 1997;11(3):359-67. PMID: 9147428.

89. Wingood GM, DiClemente RJ, Robinson-Simpson L, et al. Efficacy of an HIV intervention in reducing high-risk human papillomavirus, nonviral sexually transmitted infections, and concurrency among African American women: a randomized-controlled trial. *J Acquir Immune Defic Syndr.* 2013;63(Suppl 1):S36-43. PMID: 23673884.

90. Metsch LR, Feaster DJ, Gooden L, et al. Effect of risk-reduction counseling with rapid HIV testing on risk of acquiring sexually transmitted infections: the AWARE randomized controlled trial. *JAMA.* 2013;310(16):1701-10. PMID: 24150466.

91. Alemagno SA, Stephens RC, Stephens P, et al. Brief motivational intervention to reduce HIV risk and to increase HIV testing among offenders under community supervision. *J Correct Health Care.* 2009;15(3):210-21. PMID: 19477803.

92. Cohen DA, Dent C, MacKinnon D, et al. Condom skills education and sexually transmitted disease reinfection. *J Sex Res.* 1991;28(1):139-45.

93. Dancy BL, Dancy BL. African American adolescent females: mother-involved HIV risk-reduction intervention. *J HIV AIDS Soc Serv.* 2009;8(3):292-307. PMID: 20090855.

94. DiClemente RJ, Wingood GM, Rose E, et al. Evaluation of an HIV/STD sexual risk-reduction intervention for pregnant African American adolescents attending a prenatal clinic in an urban public hospital: preliminary evidence of efficacy. *J Pediatr Adolesc Gynecol.* 2010;23(1):32-8. PMID: 19643646.

95.   Dilley JW, Woods WJ, Sabatino J, et al. Changing sexual behavior among gay male repeat testers for HIV: a randomized, controlled trial of a single-session intervention. *J Acquir Immune Defic Syndr*. 2002;30(2):177-86.

96.   Grimley DM, Hook EW III. A 15-minute interactive, computerized condom use intervention with biological endpoints. *Sex Transm Dis*. 2009;36(2):73-8. PMID: 19125141.

97.   Howard MN, Howard MN. Improving low-income teen health behaviors with Internet-linked clinic interventions. *Sex Res Social Policy*. 2011;8(1).

98.   Lindenberg CS, Solorzano RM, Bear D, et al. Reducing substance use and risky sexual behavior among young, low-income, Mexican-American women: comparison of two interventions. *Appl Nurs Res*. 2002;15(3):137-48. PMID: 12173165.

99.   Mallory C, Hesson-McInnis M. Pilot test results of an HIV prevention intervention for high-risk women. *West J Nurs Res*. 2013;35(3):313-29. PMID: 21827425.

100.   Morrison-Beedy D, Carey MP, Kowalski J, et al. Group-based HIV risk reduction intervention for adolescent girls: evidence of feasibility and efficacy. *Res Nurs Health*. 2005;28(1):3-15. PMID: 15625713.

101.   Roye C, Perlmutter SP, Krauss B. A brief, low-cost, theory-based intervention to promote dual method use by black and Latina female adolescents: a randomized clinical trial. *Health Educ Behav*. 2007;34(4):608-21. PMID: 16740522.

102.   Senn N, de Valliere S, Berdoz D, et al. Motivational brief intervention for the prevention of sexually transmitted infections in travelers: a randomized controlled trial. *BMC Infect Dis*. 2011;11:300. PMID: 22044609.

103.   Smith PB, Weinman ML, Parrilli J. The role of condom motivation education in the reduction of new and reinfection rates of sexually transmitted diseases among inner-city female adolescents. *Patient Educ Couns*. 1997;31(1):77-81.

104.   Pealer LN, Peterman TA, Newman DR, et al. Are counselor demographics associated with successful human immunodeficiency virus/sexually transmitted disease prevention counseling? *Sex Transm Dis*. 2004;31(1):52-6. PMID: 14695958.

105.   Melendez RM, Hoffman S, Exner T, et al. Intimate partner violence and safer sex negotiation: effects of a gender-specific intervention. *Arch Sex Behav*. 2003;32(6):499-511. PMID: 14574094.

106.   DiClemente RJ, Crosby RA, Salazar LF, et al. Is male intent to be vaccinated against HPV a function of the promotion message? *Int J STD AIDS*. 2011;22(6):332-4.

107.   Eaton LA, Huedo-Medina TB, Kalichman SC, et al. Meta-analysis of single-session behavioral interventions to prevent sexually transmitted infections: implications for bundling prevention packages. *Am J Public Health*. 2012;102(11):e34-e44. PMID: 22994247.

108.   Chin HB, Sipe TA, Elder R, et al. The effectiveness of group-based comprehensive risk-reduction and abstinence education interventions to prevent or reduce the risk of adolescent pregnancy, human immunodeficiency virus, and sexually transmitted infections: two systematic reviews for the Guide to Community Preventive Services. *Am J Prev Med*. 2012;42(3):272-94. PMID: 22341164.

109.   Smoak ND, Scott-Sheldon LA, Johnson BT, et al. Sexual risk reduction interventions do not inadvertently increase the overall frequency of sexual behavior: a meta-analysis of 174 studies with 116,735 participants. *J Acquir Immune Defic Syndr*. 2006;41(3):374-84. PMID: 16540941.

110. Catania JA, Kegeles SM, Coates TJ. Towards an understanding of risk behavior: an AIDS Risk Reduction Model (ARRM). *Health Educ Q*. 1990;17(1):53-72.

111. Fisher JD, Fisher WA. Changing AIDS-risk behavior. *Psychol Bull*. 1992;111(3):455-74.

112. Lawrence JS, Fortenberry JD. Behavorial Interventions for STDs: Theoretical Models and Intervention Methods. In: Aral SO, Douglas JM Jr, Lipshutz JA (eds). Behavioral Interventions for Prevention and Control of Sexually Transmitted Diseases. Atlanta, GA: Springer; 2007. p. 23-59.

113. Noar SM. Behavioral interventions to reduce HIV-related sexual risk behavior: review and synthesis of meta-analytic evidence. *AIDS Behav*. 2008;12(3):335-53. PMID: 17896176.

114. Risser WL, Bortot AT, Benjamins LJ, et al. The epidemiology of sexually transmitted infections in adolescents. *Semin Pediatr Infect Dis*. 2005;16(3):160-7. PMID: 16044389.

115. Javanbakht M, Guerry S, Gorbach PM, et al. Prevalence and correlates of heterosexual anal intercourse among clients attending public sexually transmitted disease clinics in Los Angeles County. *Sex Transm Dis*. 2010;37(6):369-76.

116. Charania MR, Crepaz N, Guenther-Gray C, et al. Efficacy of structural-level condom distribution interventions: a meta-analysis of U.S. and international studies, 1998-2007. *AIDS Behav*. 2011;15(7):1283-97. PMID: 20886277.

117. Barker DH, Swenson RR, Brown LK, et al. Blocking the benefit of group-based HIV-prevention efforts during adolescence: the problem of HIV-related stigma. *AIDS Behav*. 2012;16(3):571-7. PMID: 22170381.

118. Hollis JF, Polen MR, Whitlock EP, et al. Teen reach: outcomes from a randomized, controlled trial of a tobacco reduction program for teens seen in primary medical care. *Pediatrics*. 2005;115(4):981-9. PMID: 15805374.

119. Rose E, DiClemente RJ, Wingood GM, et al. The validity of teens' and young adults' self-reported condom use. *Arch Pediatr Adolesc Med*. 2009;163(1):61-4.

120. Herbst JH, Beeker C, Mathew A, et al. The effectiveness of individual-, group-, and community-level HIV behavioral risk-reduction interventions for adult men who have sex with men: a systematic review. *Am J Prev Med*. 2007;32(4 Suppl):S38-67. PMID: 17386336.

121. Imrie J, Stephenson JM, Cowan FM, et al. A cognitive behavioural intervention to reduce sexually transmitted infections among gay men: randomised trial. *BMJ*. 2001;322(7300):1451-6.

122. Semaan S, Des Jarlais DC, Sogolow E, et al. A meta-analysis of the effect of HIV prevention interventions on the sex behaviors of drug users in the United States. *J Acquir Immune Defic Syndr*. 2002;30(Suppl 1):S73-93.

123. Meader N, Semaan S, Halton M, et al. An international systematic review and meta-analysis of multisession psychosocial interventions compared with educational or minimal interventions on the HIV sex risk behaviors of people who use drugs. *AIDS Behav*. 2013;17(6):1963-78. PMID: 23386132.

124. Shepherd J, Kavanagh J, Picot J, et al. The effectiveness and cost-effectiveness of behavioural interventions for the prevention of sexually transmitted infections in young people aged 13-19: a systematic review and economic evaluation. *Health Technol Assess*. 2010;14(7):1-206. PMID: 20178696.

125. Centers for Disease Control and Prevention. Compendium of Evidence-Based HIV Behavioral Interventions. Atlanta, GA: Centers for Disease Control and Prevention; 2013.

126. Jones R, Hoover DR, Lacroix LJ. A randomized controlled trial of soap opera videos streamed to smartphones to reduce risk of sexually transmitted human immunodeficiency virus (HIV) in young urban African American women. *Nurs Outlook.* 2013;61(4):205-15. PMID: 23743482.

127. American Academy of Family Physicians. Summary of Recommendations for Clinical Preventive Services. Leawood, KS: American Academy of Family Physicians; 2012.

128. Condom use by adolescents. *Pediatrics.* 2013;132(5):973-81.

129. Committee Opinion No. 460: the initial reproductive health visit. *Obstet Gynecol.* 2010;116(1):240-3. PMID: 20567198.

130. Committee Opinion No. 534: well-woman visit. *Obstet Gynecol.* 2012;120(2 Pt 1):421-4. PMID: 22825111.

131. ACOG Committee Opinion No. 423: motivational interviewing: a tool for behavioral change. *Obstet Gynecol.* 2009;113(1):243-6. PMID: 19104391.

132. ACOG Committee Opinion No. 525: health care for lesbians and bisexual women. *Obstet Gynecol.* 2012;119(5):1077-80. PMID: 22525932.

133. ACOG Committee Opinion No. 536: human immunodeficiency virus and acquired immunodeficiency syndrome and women of color. *Obstet Gynecol.* 2012;120(3):735-9. PMID: 22914493.

134. ACOG Committee Opinion No. 582: addressing health risks of noncoital sexual activity. *Obstet Gynecol.* 2013;122(6):1378-82. PMID: 24264716.

135. Centers for Disease Control and Prevention. Sexually Transmitted Diseases Treatment Guidelines. Atlanta, GA: Centers for Disease Control and Prevention; 2010.

136. Centers for Disease Control and Prevention. HIV Infection: Detection, Counseling, and Referral. Atlanta, GA: Centers for Disease Control and Prevention; 2010.

137. Wilkinson J, Bass C, Diem S, et al. Preventive Services for Children and Adolescents. Bloomington, MN: Institute for Clinical Systems Improvement; 2013.

138. Wilkinson J, Bass C, Diem S, et al. Preventive Services for Adults. Bloomington, MN: Institute for Clinical Systems Improvement; 2013.

139. Michigan Quality Improvement Consortium. Routine Preventive Services for Children and Adolescents (Ages 2–21). Southfield, MI: Michigan Quality Improvement Consortium; 2011.

140. Allen J, Bharel M, Brammer S, et al. Adapting Your Practice: Treatment and Recommendations on Reproductive Health Care for Homeless Patients. Nashville, TN: Health Care for the Homeless Clinicians' Network, National Health Care for the Homeless Council; 2008.

141. National Institute for Health and Care Excellence. One to One Interventions to Reduce the Transmission of Sexually Transmitted Infections (STIs) Including HIV, and to Reduce the Rate of Under 18 Conceptions, Especially Among Vulnerable and at Risk Groups. London: National Institute for Health and Care Excellence; 2007.

142. University of Michigan Health System. Adult Clinical Preventive Care. Ann Arbor, MI: University of Michigan; 2011.

143. Akers DD. ASSESS: for adolescent risk reduction. In: Card JJ, Benner TA (eds). Model Programs for Adolescent Sexual Health: Evidence-Based HIV, STI, and Pregnancy Prevention Interventions. New York: Springer; 2008. p. 375-82.

144. Gottlieb SL, Douglas JM Jr, Foster M, et al. Incidence of herpes simplex virus type 2 infection in 5 sexually transmitted disease (STD) clinics and the effect of HIV/STD risk-reduction counseling. *J Infect Dis*. 2004;190(6):1059-67. PMID: 15319854.

145. Bolu OO, Lindsey C, Kamb ML, et al. Is HIV/sexually transmitted disease prevention counseling effective among vulnerable populations? A subset analysis of data collected for a randomized, controlled trial evaluating counseling efficacy (Project RESPECT). *Sex Transm Dis*. 2004;31(8):469-74. PMID: 15273579.

146. Semaan S, Neumann MS, Hutchins K, et al. Brief counseling for reducing sexual risk and bacterial STIs among drug users--results from Project RESPECT. *Drug Alcohol Depend*. 2010;106(1):7-15. PMID: 19720471.

147. Rhodes F, Stein JA, Fishbein M, et al. Using theory to understand how interventions work: Project RESPECT, condom use, and the Integrative Model. *AIDS Behav*. 2007;11(3):393-407. PMID: 17323123.

148. Benner TA. SiHLE: health workshops for young black women. In: Card JJ, Benner TA (eds). Model Programs for Adolescent Sexual Health: Evidence-Based HIV, STI and Pregnancy Prevention Interventions. New York: Springer; 2008. p. 253-60.

149. Lang DL, DiClemente RJ, Hardin JW, et al. Threats of cross-contamination on effects of a sexual risk reduction intervention: fact or fiction. *Prev Sci*. 2009;10(3):270-5. PMID: 19241171.

150. Kirby D. An HIV-prevention intervention for African American adolescent girls significantly increased condom use. *Evid Based Obstet Gynecol*. 2005;7:74-5.

151. Wingood GM, DiClemente RJ, Harrington KF, et al. Efficacy of an HIV prevention program among female adolescents experiencing gender-based violence. *Am J Public Health*. 2006;96(6):1085-90. PMID: 16670238.

152. Sales JM, Lang DL, Hardin JW, et al. Efficacy of an HIV prevention program among African American female adolescents reporting high depressive symptomatology. *J Womens Health (Larchmt)*. 2010;19(2):219-27. PMID: 20109119.

153. Milhausen RR, DiClemente RJ, Lang DL, et al. Frequency of sex after an intervention to decrease sexual risk-taking among African-American adolescent girls: results of a randomized, controlled clinical trial. *Sex Educ*. 2008;8:47-57.

154. Korte JE, Shain RN, Holden AE, et al. Reduction in sexual risk behaviors and infection rates among African Americans and Mexican Americans. *Sex Transm Dis*. 2004;31(3):166-73. PMID: 15076930.

155. Thurman AR, Holden AE, Shain RN, et al. Preventing recurrent sexually transmitted diseases in minority adolescents: a randomized controlled trial. *Obstet Gynecol*. 2008;111(6):1417-25. PMID: 18515527.

156. Holden AE, Shain RN, Miller WB, et al. The influence of depression on sexual risk reduction and STD infection in a controlled, randomized intervention trial. *Sex Transm Dis*. 2008;35(10):898-904. PMID: 18607311.

157. Carey MP, Vanable PA, Senn TE, et al. Evaluating a two-step approach to sexual risk reduction in a publicly-funded STI clinic: rationale, design, and baseline data from the Health Improvement Project-Rochester (HIP-R). *Contemp Clin Trials*. 2008;29(4):569-86. PMID: 18325853.

158. Mittal M, Senn TE, Carey MP. Mediators of the relation between partner violence and sexual risk behavior among women attending a sexually transmitted disease clinic. *Sex Transm Dis.* 2011;38(6):510-5. PMID: 21258269.

159. Peipert J, Redding CA, Blume J, et al. Design of a stage-matched intervention trial to increase dual method contraceptive use (Project PROTECT). *Contemp Clin Trials.* 2007;28(5):626-37. PMID: 17374567.

160. O'Leary A, Jemmott LS, Jemmott JB. Mediation analysis of an effective sexual risk-reduction intervention for women: the importance of self-efficacy. *Health Psychol.* 2008;27(2 Suppl):S180-4. PMID: 18377160.

161. Marrazzo JM, Thomas KK, Fiedler TL, et al. Relationship of specific vaginal bacteria and bacterial vaginosis treatment failure in women who have sex with women. *Ann Intern Med.* 2008;149(1):20-8. PMID: 18591634.

162. Marrazzo JM, Thomas KK, Agnew K, et al. Prevalence and risks for bacterial vaginosis in women who have sex with women. *Sex Transm Dis.* 2010;37(5):335-9. PMID: 20429087.

163. Hoffman S, Exner TM, Leu CS, et al. Female-condom use in a gender-specific family planning clinic trial. *Am J Public Health.* 2003;93(11):1897-903. PMID: 14600063.

164. Enrhardt AA, Exner TM, Hoffman S, et al. HIV/STD risk and sexual strategies among women family planning clients in New York: Project FIO. *AIDS Behav.* 2002;6(1):1-13.

165. Miller S, Exner TM, Williams SP, et al. A gender-specific intervention for at-risk women in the USA. *AIDS Care.* 2000;12(5):603-12. PMID: 11218546.

166. Dworkin SL, Beckford ST, Ehrhardt AA. Sexual scripts of women: a longitudinal analysis of participants in a gender-specific HIV/STD prevention intervention. *Arch Sex Behav.* 2007;36(2):269-79. PMID: 17186128.

167. Champion JD. Behavioural interventions and abuse: secondary analysis of reinfection in minority women. *Int J STD AIDS.* 2007;18(11):748-53. PMID: 18005508.

168. Arnold EA. A Randomized Controlled Trial of the Bruthas Project. San Francisco, CA: University of California, San Francisco; 2012. Accessed at http://clinicaltrials.gov/ct2/show/NCT01270230?term=Bruthas&rank=1 on 15 September 2014.

169. Brady S. HIV Prevention With the Mentally Ill. Boston, MA: Boston Medical Center; 2010. Accessed at http://clinicaltrials.gov/ct2/show/NCT00643305?term=HIV+prevention+mentally+ill&rank=1 on 14 September 2014.

170. Brady S. HIV/AIDS, Severe Mental Illness and Homelessness. Boston, MA: Boston University; 2012. Accessed at http://clinicaltrials.gov/ct2/show/NCT01172704?term=HIV%2FAIDS+mental+illness&rank=1 on 15 September 2014.

171. Bull S. Effectiveness of an Online Prevention Program in Reducing the Risk of STD Infection in Young Adults (Youthnet). Denver, CO: University of Colorado, Denver; 2008. Accessed at http://clinicaltrials.gov/ct2/show/NCT00255944?term=youthnet&rank=2 on 15 September 2014.

172. Colfax GN. Reducing HIV Risk Among Episodic Substance Using Men Who Have Sex With Men. San Francisco, CA: HIV Prevention Section, San Francisco Department of Public Health; 2011. Accessed at http://clinicaltrials.gov/ct2/show/NCT01279044?term=reducing+HIV&rank=6 on 15 September 2014.

173. Crosby RA, Mena LA. Safer Sex Program for Young African-American Men. Lexington, KY: University of Kentucky; 2012. Accessed at http://clinicaltrials.gov/ct2/show/NCT01439503?term=safer+sex+program&rank=1 on 15 September 2014.

174. DiClemente RJ. HIV Prevention for African American Teens. Atlanta, GA: Emory University; 2012. Accessed at http://clinicaltrials.gov/ct2/show/NCT00279799?term=Afiya&rank=1 on 15 September 2014.

175. Du Bois SN, Johnson SE, Mustanski B. Examining racial and ethnic minority differences among YMSM during recruitment for an online HIV prevention intervention study. *AIDS Behav.* 2012;16(6):1430-5. PMID: 21986869.

176. Fernandez I. Proyecto SOL: A Risk Reduction Intervention for Hispanic Men Who Have Sex With Men. Fort Lauderdale, FL: Nova Southeastern University; 2010. Accessed at http://clinicaltrials.gov/ct2/show/NCT00690976?term=proyecto+SOL&rank=1 on 15 September 2014.

177. Garofalo R. HIV Prevention Intervention for Young Transgender Women (LifeSkills). Chicago, IL: Ann & Robert H. Lurie Children's Hospital of Chicago; 2012. Accessed at http://clinicaltrials.gov/ct2/show/NCT01575938?term=LifeSkills&rank=2 on 15 September 2014.

178. Gold MA. The S.A.F.E. Study: Computer-Aided Counseling to Prevent Teen Pregnancy/Sexually Transmitted Diseases (STDs). Pittsburgh, Pennsylvania: University of Pittsburgh; 2011. Accessed at http://clinicaltrials.gov/ct2/show/NCT00151151?term=S.A.F.E.&rank=2 on 15 September 2014.

179. Houck CD. Affect Management for Early Adolescents. Providence, RI: Rhode Island Hospital; 2012. Accessed at http://clinicaltrials.gov/ct2/show/NCT01197404?term=affect+management&rank=1 on 15 September 2014.

180. Ickovics J. Group Prenatal Care for Reducing the Risk of STDs in Pregnant Young Women. New Haven, CT: Yale University; 2012. Accessed at http://clinicaltrials.gov/ct2/show/NCT00271960?term=prenatal+care+for+reducing&rank=1 on 15 September 2014.

181. Kapungu CT, Kapungu CT. Recruiting and retaining high-risk adolescents into family-based HIV prevention intervention research. *J Child Fam Studies.* 2012;21(4).

182. Lauby JL. Evaluation of a New HIV Prevention Intervention for Black Bisexually-Active Men. Philadelphia, PA: Public Health Management Corporation; 2011. Accessed at http://clinicaltrials.gov/ct2/show/NCT01347164?term=bisexually-active&rank=1 on 15 September 2014.

183. Llewellyn C, Abraham C, Miners A, et al. Multicentre RCT and economic evaluation of a psychological intervention together with a leaflet to reduce risk behaviour amongst men who have sex with men (MSM) prescribed post-exposure prophylaxis for HIV following sexual exposure (PEPSE): a protocol. *BMC Infect Dis*. 2012;12:70. PMID: 22440090.

184. Lescano C. Randomized Controlled Trial of Family-Based HIV Prevention for Latinos (Latino STYLE). Tampa, FL: University of South Florida; 2012. Accessed at http://clinicaltrials.gov/ct2/show/NCT01635335?term=Latino+STYLE&rank=1 on 15 September 2014.

185. Miller LC. Effectiveness of Interactive Virtual Environment Games in Reducing Risky Sexual Behavior Among Men Who Have Sex With Men (the SOLVE-IT Study). Los Angeles, CA: University of Southern California; 2009. Accessed at http://clinicaltrials.gov/ct2/show/NCT00653991?term=SOLVE-IT&rank=1 on 15 September 2014.

186. Morokoff P. Increasing Condom Use in People at Risk for HIV Infection. Providence, RI: University of Rhode Island; 2008. Accessed at http://clinicaltrials.gov/ct2/show/NCT00080093?term=morokoff&rank=1 on 15 September 2014.

187. Murphy DA. Family-Based HIV Prevention for Adolescent Girls. Los Angeles, CA: University of California, Los Angeles; 2011. Accessed at http://clinicaltrials.gov/ct2/show/NCT00243126?term=family-based+hiv+prevention+for+adolescent+girls&rank=1 on 15 September 2014.

188. Noar SM. Computerized HIV/Sexually Transmitted Disease (STD) Prevention Program (TIPSS). Lexington, KY: University of Kentucky; 2011. Accessed at http://clinicaltrials.gov/ct2/show/NCT00947947?term=tipss&rank=1 on 15 September 2014.

189. Noar SM, Webb EM, Van Stee SK, et al. Using computer technology for HIV Prevention among African-Americans: development of a tailored information program for safer sex (TIPSS). *Health Educ Res*. 2011;26(3):393-406. PMID: 21257676.

190. O'Donnell L. No Excuses/Sin Buscar Excusas Intervention to Reduce Latino Men's HIV Risks. New York, NY: Education Development Center; 2010. Accessed at http://clinicaltrials.gov/ct2/show/NCT00690690?term=no+excuses&rank=1 on 15 September 2014.

191. Patterson TL. STD Risk Reduction for Heterosexual Methamphetamine Users. San Diego, CA: University of California, San Diego; 2012. Accessed at http://clinicaltrials.gov/ct2/show/NCT00344214?term=std+risk+reduction+for+methamphetamine&rank=1 on 15 September 2014.

192. Rizzo CJ. Dating Violence and HIV Prevention for Girls: Adapting Mental Health Interventions. Providence, RI: Rhode Island Hospital; 2012. Accessed at http://clinicaltrials.gov/ct2/show/NCT01326195?term=adapting+mental+health+interventions&rank=1 on 15 September 2014.

193. Shegog R, Markham C, Peskin M, Et Al. Internet-Based Sexual Health Education for Middle School Native American Youth. Houston, TX: University of Texas Health Science Center; 2011. Accessed at http://clinicaltrials.gov/ct2/show/NCT01303575?term=iyg-ai%2fan&rank=1 on 15 September 2014.

194. Sperling C. An STD Prevention Intervention for Men Newly Released From Jail. Decatur, GA: STAND; 2012. Accessed at http://clinicaltrials.gov/ct2/show/NCT00260780?term=misters&rank=2 on 15 September 2014.
195. Sullivan LE. Reducing Sex-Related HIV Risk Behaviors in Patients Receiving Treatment for Opioid Dependence (Project RED). New Haven, CT: Yale University; 2010. Accessed at http://clinicaltrials.gov/ct2/show/NCT00548275?term=project+red&rank=1 on 15 September 2014.
196. University Of Pittsburgh. Text-Message Program to Reduce Risk Sexual Behaviors in Young Adult Female Emergency Department Patients (STARSS). Pittsburgh, PA: University of Pittsburgh; 2012. Accessed at http://clinicaltrials.gov/ct2/show/NCT01548183?term=starss&rank=1 on 15 September 2014.
197. Wechsberg WM. Young Women's COOP Study. Durham, NC: Research Triangle Institute International; 2012. Accessed at http://clinicaltrials.gov/ct2/show/NCT01224184?term=coop&rank=2 on 15 September 2014.
198. Wu E. Connect 'N Unite: Couples-Based HIV/STI Prevention for Drug-Involved, Black MSM. New York, NY: Columbia University; 2012. Accessed at http://clinicaltrials.gov/ct2/show/NCT01394900?term=connect+%27n&rank=1 on 15 September 2014.
199. Zule W. Computer-Assisted Tailored Cue-Card Health (CATCH) Study. Durham, NC: Research Triangle Institute International; 2011. Accessed at http://clinicaltrials.gov/ct2/show/NCT01170741?term=catch&rank=3 on 15 September 2014.

Figure 1. Analytic Framework

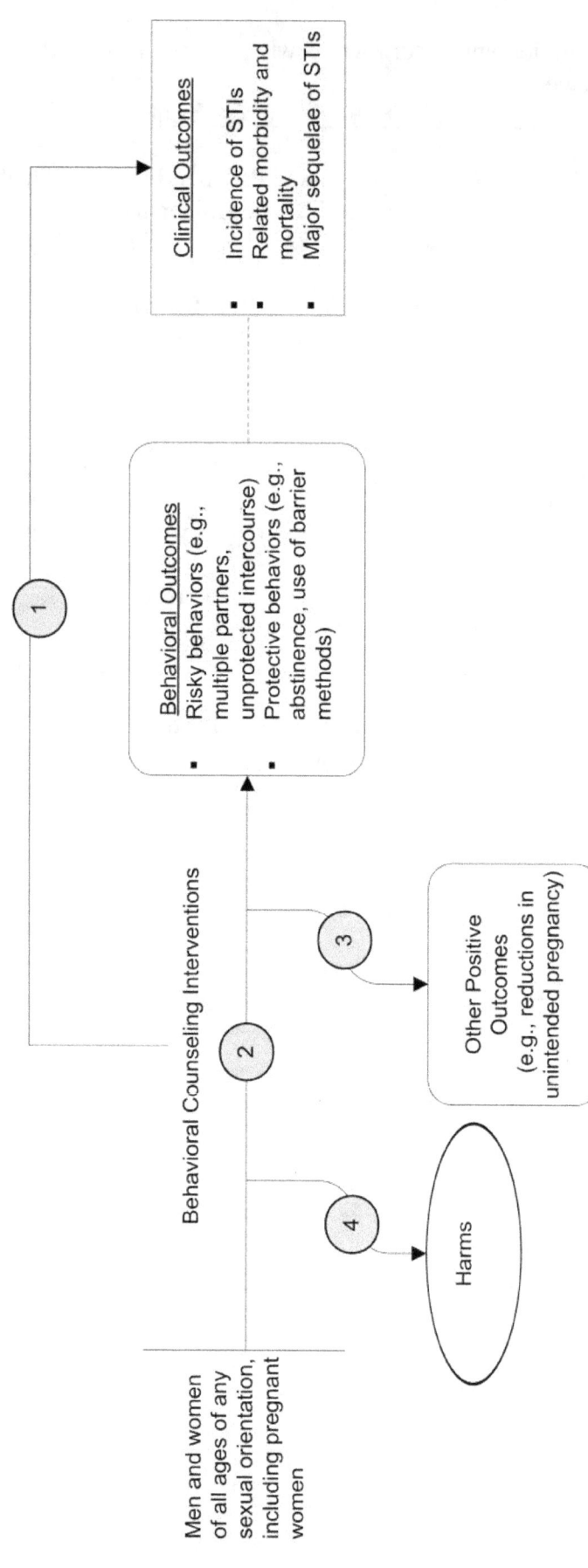

Abbreviation: STI = sexually transmitted infection.

Figure 2. Included Trials, by Intervention Intensity and Population Risk, Showing the Primary Outcome and Noting Trials With Narrowly Targeted Samples

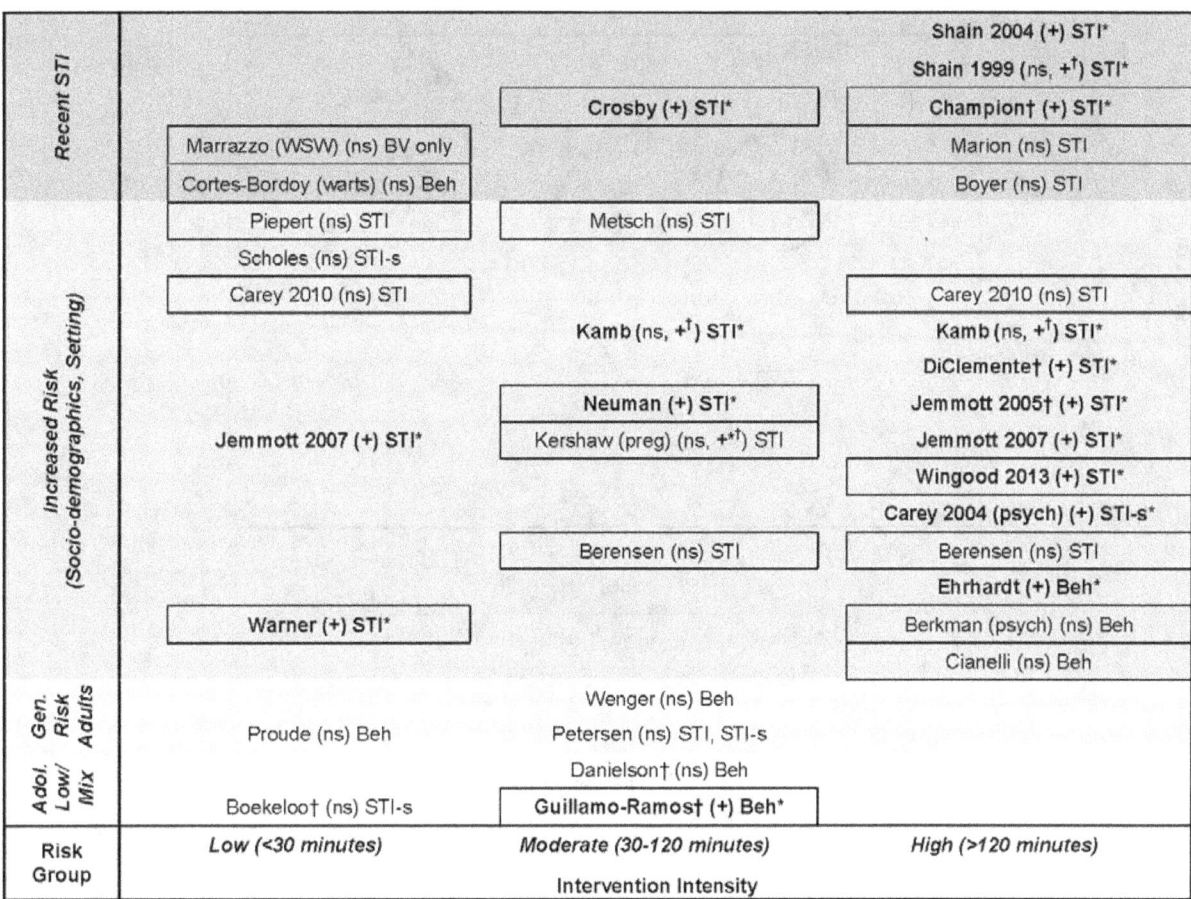

*Statistically significant group differences in primary outcome (**bolded**).
†Adolescents only.
‡Outlined studies indicate new studies added since the 2008 USPSTF review.

Abbreviations: adol = adolescents; Beh = primary outcome was a behavioral outcome; BV = only STI reported was bacterial vaginosis; Gen = general; ns = not significant; preg = trials limited to pregnant women; psych = trials limited to psychiatric patients; STI = reported sexually transmitted infection outcome; WSW = trial limited to women who have sex with women.

Figure 3. Distribution of Included Studies Across the Levels of Treatment Intensity and Population Risk, Weighted by Sample Size

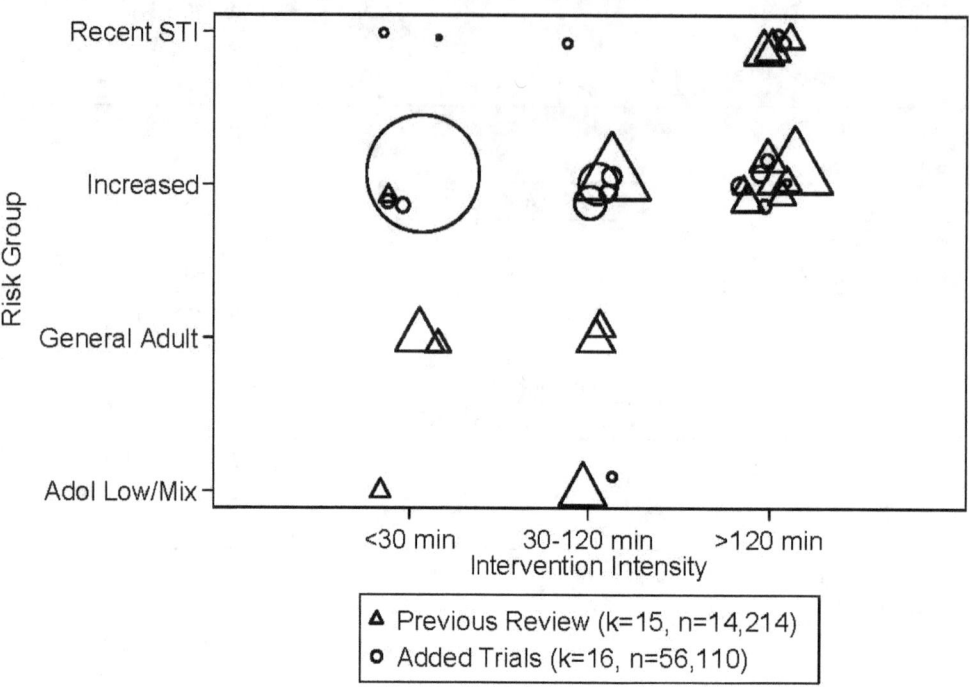

Abbreviations: adol = adolescents; min = minute(s); STI = sexually transmitted infection.

Figure 4. Forest Plot of STI Incidence in Included Trials Targeting Adolescents

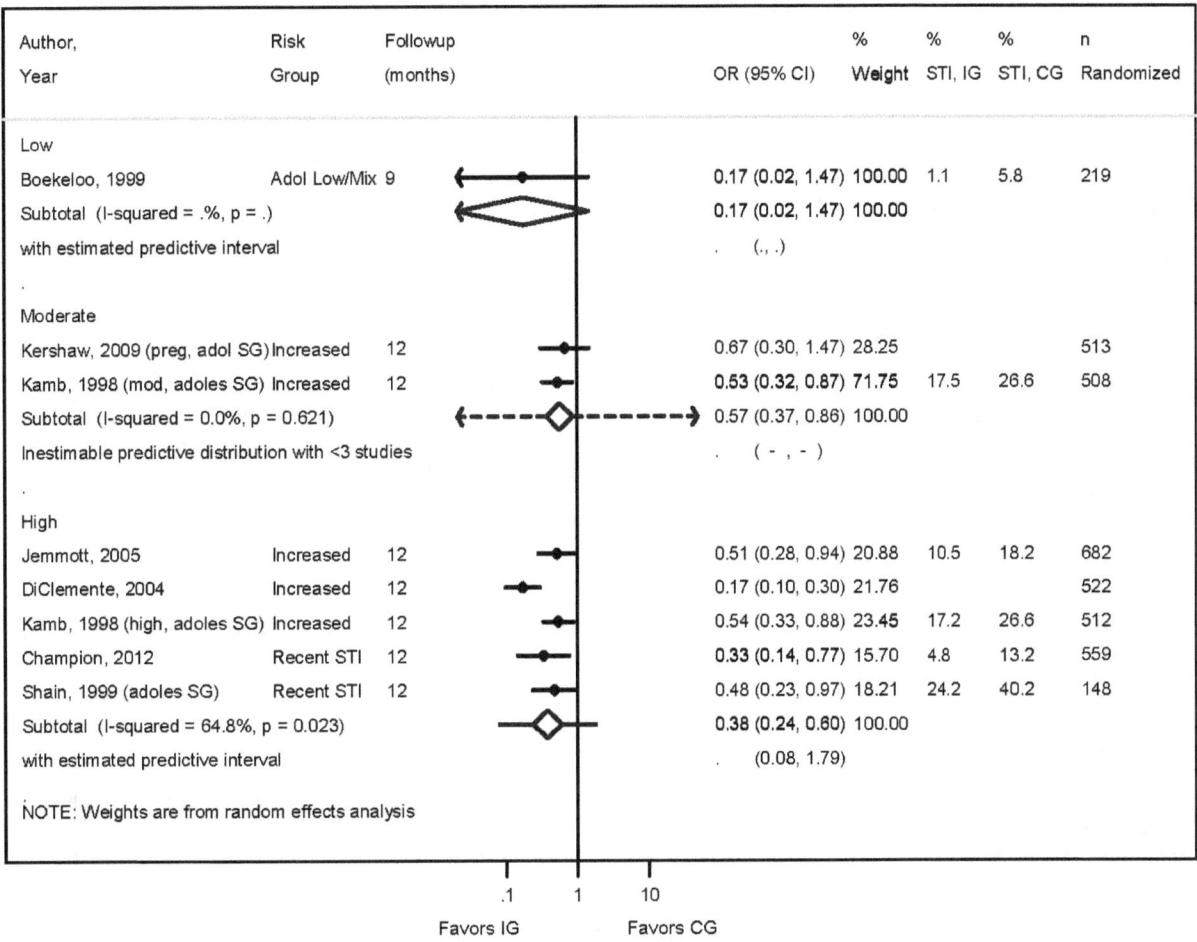

Author, Year	Risk Group	Followup (months)	OR (95% CI)	% Weight	% STI, IG	% STI, CG	n Randomized
Low							
Boekeloo, 1999	Adol Low/Mix	9	0.17 (0.02, 1.47)	100.00	1.1	5.8	219
Subtotal (I-squared = .%, p = .)			0.17 (0.02, 1.47)	100.00			
with estimated predictive interval			. (., .)				
Moderate							
Kershaw, 2009 (preg, adol SG)	Increased	12	0.67 (0.30, 1.47)	28.25			513
Kamb, 1998 (mod, adoles SG)	Increased	12	0.53 (0.32, 0.87)	71.75	17.5	26.6	508
Subtotal (I-squared = 0.0%, p = 0.621)			0.57 (0.37, 0.86)	100.00			
Inestimable predictive distribution with <3 studies			. (- , -)				
High							
Jemmott, 2005	Increased	12	0.51 (0.28, 0.94)	20.88	10.5	18.2	682
DiClemente, 2004	Increased	12	0.17 (0.10, 0.30)	21.76			522
Kamb, 1998 (high, adoles SG)	Increased	12	0.54 (0.33, 0.88)	23.45	17.2	26.6	512
Champion, 2012	Recent STI	12	0.33 (0.14, 0.77)	15.70	4.8	13.2	559
Shain, 1999 (adoles SG)	Recent STI	12	0.48 (0.23, 0.97)	18.21	24.2	40.2	148
Subtotal (I-squared = 64.8%, p = 0.023)			0.38 (0.24, 0.60)	100.00			
with estimated predictive interval			. (0.08, 1.79)				

NOTE: Weights are from random effects analysis

.1   1   10

Favors IG   Favors CG

Abbreviations: adol/es = adolescent; CG = control group; CI = confidence interval; IG = intervention group; mod = moderate intensity; OR = odds ratio; preg = pregnant; SG = subgroup; STI = sexually transmitted infection.

Figure 5. Forest Plot of STI Incidence in Included Trials Targeting Adults

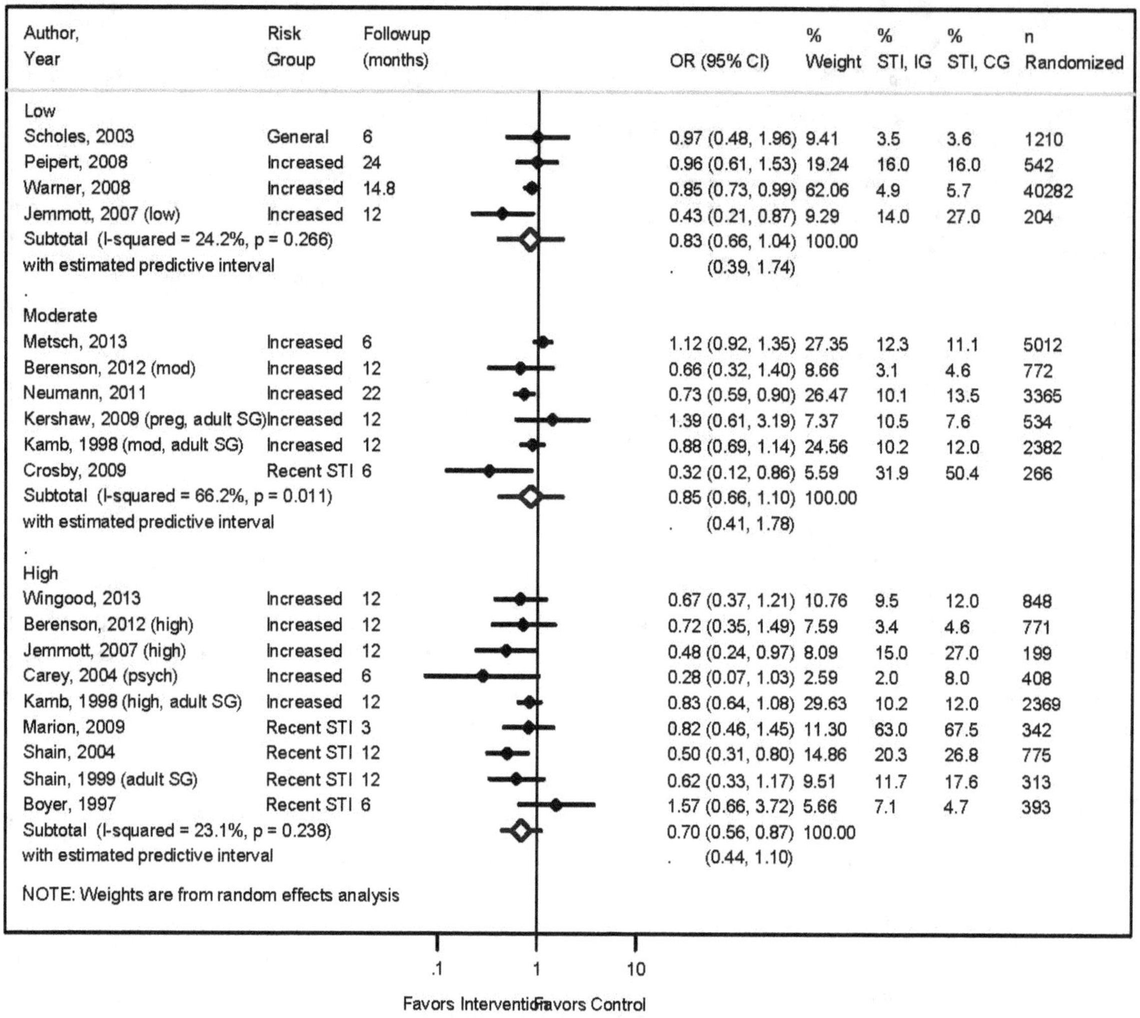

Author, Year	Risk Group	Followup (months)	OR (95% CI)	% Weight	% STI, IG	% STI, CG	n Randomized
Low							
Scholes, 2003	General	6	0.97 (0.48, 1.96)	9.41	3.5	3.6	1210
Peipert, 2008	Increased	24	0.96 (0.61, 1.53)	19.24	16.0	16.0	542
Warner, 2008	Increased	14.8	0.85 (0.73, 0.99)	62.06	4.9	5.7	40282
Jemmott, 2007 (low)	Increased	12	0.43 (0.21, 0.87)	9.29	14.0	27.0	204
Subtotal (I-squared = 24.2%, p = 0.266)			0.83 (0.66, 1.04)	100.00			
with estimated predictive interval			(0.39, 1.74)				
Moderate							
Metsch, 2013	Increased	6	1.12 (0.92, 1.35)	27.35	12.3	11.1	5012
Berenson, 2012 (mod)	Increased	12	0.66 (0.32, 1.40)	8.66	3.1	4.6	772
Neumann, 2011	Increased	22	0.73 (0.59, 0.90)	26.47	10.1	13.5	3365
Kershaw, 2009 (preg, adult SG)	Increased	12	1.39 (0.61, 3.19)	7.37	10.5	7.6	534
Kamb, 1998 (mod, adult SG)	Increased	12	0.88 (0.69, 1.14)	24.56	10.2	12.0	2382
Crosby, 2009	Recent STI	6	0.32 (0.12, 0.86)	5.59	31.9	50.4	266
Subtotal (I-squared = 66.2%, p = 0.011)			0.85 (0.66, 1.10)	100.00			
with estimated predictive interval			(0.41, 1.78)				
High							
Wingood, 2013	Increased	12	0.67 (0.37, 1.21)	10.76	9.5	12.0	848
Berenson, 2012 (high)	Increased	12	0.72 (0.35, 1.49)	7.59	3.4	4.6	771
Jemmott, 2007 (high)	Increased	12	0.48 (0.24, 0.97)	8.09	15.0	27.0	199
Carey, 2004 (psych)	Increased	6	0.28 (0.07, 1.03)	2.59	2.0	8.0	408
Kamb, 1998 (high, adult SG)	Increased	12	0.83 (0.64, 1.08)	29.63	10.2	12.0	2369
Marion, 2009	Recent STI	3	0.82 (0.46, 1.45)	11.30	63.0	67.5	342
Shain, 2004	Recent STI	12	0.50 (0.31, 0.80)	14.86	20.3	26.8	775
Shain, 1999 (adult SG)	Recent STI	12	0.62 (0.33, 1.17)	9.51	11.7	17.6	313
Boyer, 1997	Recent STI	6	1.57 (0.66, 3.72)	5.66	7.1	4.7	393
Subtotal (I-squared = 23.1%, p = 0.238)			0.70 (0.56, 0.87)	100.00			
with estimated predictive interval			(0.44, 1.10)				

NOTE: Weights are from random effects analysis

.1   1   10

Favors Intervention   Favors Control

Abbreviations: CG = control group; CI = confidence interval; IG = intervention group; mod = moderate intensity; OR = odds ratio; preg = pregnant; psych = psychiatric patients; SG = subgroup; STI = sexually transmitted infection.

Figure 6. Forest Plot of Condom Use and Unprotected Sexual Intercourse in Included Trials Targeting Adults

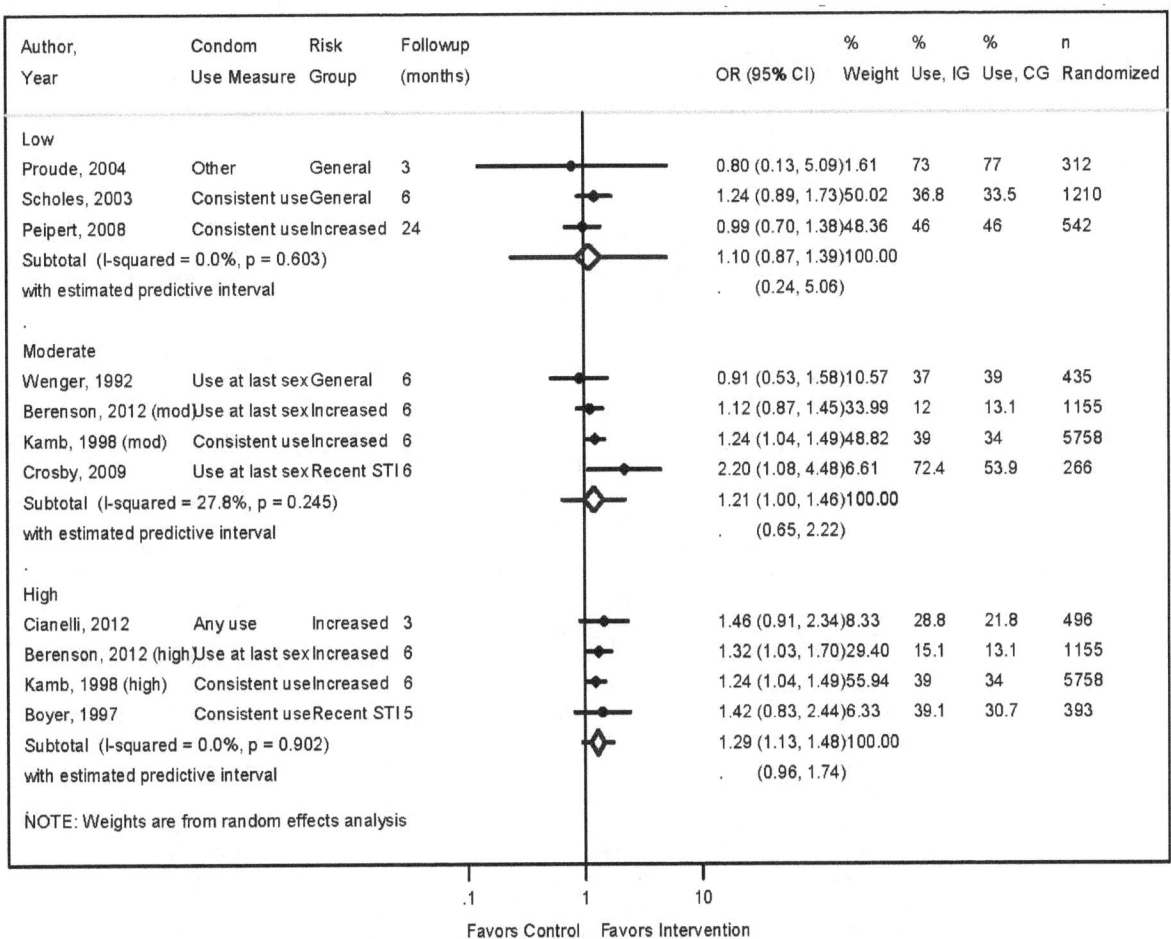

Author, Year	Condom Use Measure	Risk Group	Followup (months)	OR (95% CI)	% Weight	% Use, IG	% Use, CG	n Randomized
Low								
Proude, 2004	Other	General	3	0.80 (0.13, 5.09)	1.61	73	77	312
Scholes, 2003	Consistent use	General	6	1.24 (0.89, 1.73)	50.02	36.8	33.5	1210
Peipert, 2008	Consistent use	Increased	24	0.99 (0.70, 1.38)	48.36	46	46	542
Subtotal (I-squared = 0.0%, p = 0.603)				1.10 (0.87, 1.39)	100.00			
with estimated predictive interval				(0.24, 5.06)				
Moderate								
Wenger, 1992	Use at last sex	General	6	0.91 (0.53, 1.58)	10.57	37	39	435
Berenson, 2012 (mod)	Use at last sex	Increased	6	1.12 (0.87, 1.45)	33.99	12	13.1	1155
Kamb, 1998 (mod)	Consistent use	Increased	6	1.24 (1.04, 1.49)	48.82	39	34	5758
Crosby, 2009	Use at last sex	Recent STI	6	2.20 (1.08, 4.48)	6.61	72.4	53.9	266
Subtotal (I-squared = 27.8%, p = 0.245)				1.21 (1.00, 1.46)	100.00			
with estimated predictive interval				(0.65, 2.22)				
High								
Cianelli, 2012	Any use	Increased	3	1.46 (0.91, 2.34)	8.33	28.8	21.8	496
Berenson, 2012 (high)	Use at last sex	Increased	6	1.32 (1.03, 1.70)	29.40	15.1	13.1	1155
Kamb, 1998 (high)	Consistent use	Increased	6	1.24 (1.04, 1.49)	55.94	39	34	5758
Boyer, 1997	Consistent use	Recent STI	5	1.42 (0.83, 2.44)	6.33	39.1	30.7	393
Subtotal (I-squared = 0.0%, p = 0.902)				1.29 (1.13, 1.48)	100.00			
with estimated predictive interval				(0.96, 1.74)				

NOTE: Weights are from random effects analysis

.1   1   10

Favors Control   Favors Intervention

Abbreviations: CG = control group; CI = confidence interval; IG = intervention group; OR = odds ratio; STI = sexually transmitted infection.

Table 1. Recommendations of Other Organizations for Sexual Risk Reduction Counseling to Prevent STIs

Organization, Year	Recommendation
American Academy of Family Physicians (AAFP), 2012	AAFP recommends high-intensity behavioral counseling to prevent STIs in all sexually active adolescents and high-risk adults.[127] It concludes that the current evidence is insufficient to assess the benefits and harms of behavioral counseling to prevent STIs in presexually active adolescents and in adults not at increased risk for STIs. These recommendations were based on the USPSTF 2008 recommendation statement.
American Academy of Pediatrics (AAP), 2013	AAP targets several recommendations to pediatricians and other clinicians, including 1) clinicians should actively support and encourage the consistent and correct use of condoms as part of anticipatory guidance in adolescents; 2) clinicians should promote communication between parents and adolescents about healthy sexual development and effective use of condoms; 3) clinicians should raise awareness that making condoms available does not increase the onset or frequency of adolescent sexual activity; 4) clinicians should provide and support parental education programs to help parents develop communication skills with their adolescent children around preventions of STIs and proper use of condoms.[128]
American Congress of Obstetricians and Gynecologists (ACOG), 2008-2013	ACOG recommends discussing contraception and STIs during adolescents' initial reproductive health visits and provides time-based coding recommendations for individual counseling in preventive medicine, risk factor reduction, or both in individuals without a specific illness to promote health and prevention, illness or injury, or both.[129] It recognizes that the annual well-woman visit provides an excellent opportunity to counsel patients about maintaining a healthy lifestyle and minimizing health risks, and it should include screening, evaluation and counseling, and immunizations based on the patient's age and risk factors.[130] Applying principles of motivational interviewing (e.g., prompting patients to use safe sex practices and to use contraception more consistently) to daily patient practices has been proved effective in eliciting behavior change that contributes to positive health outcomes and improved patient-physician communication.[131] Among lesbian and bisexual patients, comprehensive care including prevention of STIs is recommended.[132] Education about the risks for STIs and dispelling the perception that transmission of STIs between women is negligible will help patients make informed decisions. All patients should be encouraged to use safe sex practices to reduce the risk for transmitting or acquiring STIs and HIV, such as using condoms on sex toys, gloves, and dental dams, as well as avoidance of sharing other sex paraphernalia. Among women of color, several approaches (e.g., gender-tailored and culturally appropriate interventions to reduce risk-taking behavior) can reduce the rate of HIV infection and optimize health.[133] For women participating in noncoital activities, clinicians should assess the patient's STI risk and provide risk reduction counseling.[134] When engaging in oral and anal sex, most individuals, including adolescents, are unlikely to use barrier protection for a variety of reasons, including a greater perceived safety compared with vaginal sex. Clinicians should encourage and counsel patients in the correct and consistent use of condoms, barrier protection during oral sex, and cleaning of sex toys.
Centers for Disease Control and Prevention (CDC), 2010	The CDC recommends that all providers should routinely obtain a sexual history from their patients and encourage risk reduction using various strategies (e.g., prevention counseling).[135] It also recommends that HIV prevention counseling should be offered and encouraged in all health care facilities that serve patients at high risk (e.g., STI clinics).[136]
Institute for Clinical Systems Improvement (ICSI), 2013	For children and adolecents, counseling regarding sexual behaviors to prevent STIs could be recommended beginning at age 12 (Weak Recommendation).[137] There is good evidence that behavioral counseling involving multiple-visit interventions is effective in reducing the incidence of STIs for sexually active adolescents. There is insufficient evidence to show efficacy for less intense interventions and low-risk patients. For adults, counseling regarding sexual behaviors to prevent STIs by clinicians and health care systems could be recommended (Weak Recommendation). ICSI concludes there is good evidence that behavioral counseling involving multiple-visit interventions is effective in reducing the incidence of STIs for higher-risk adults. There is insufficient evidence to show efficacy for less intense interventions and low-risk patients.[138] Both recommendations are Level III preventive services.
Michigan Quality Improvement Consortium (MQIC), 2011	MQIC recommends parent and child age-appropriate education and counseling to prevent STIs among all children and adolescents ages 2 to 21 years.[139]
National Health Care for the Homeless Council, 2008	The National Health Care for the Homeless Council recommends counseling at-risk clients to adopt safer sexual behavior to prevent STIs (e.g., use of interactive counseling that focuses on preventing unwanted pregnancy and transmission of disease).[140]

Table 1. Recommendations of Other Organizations for Sexual Risk Reduction Counseling to Prevent STIs

Organization, Year	Recommendation
National Institute for Health and Care Excellence (NICE), 2007	After identifying individuals at high risk for STIs, NICE recommends having one-to-one structured discussions with these individuals (if the health professional is trained in sexual health) or arranging for these discussions to take place with a trained practitioner.[141] Among vulnerable young people younger than age 18 years, including pregnant women and mothers, when appropriate, practitioners should provide one-to-one sexual advice on how to prevent and/or get tested for STIs.
University of Michigan Health System (UMHS), 2011	UMHS recommends intensive STI counseling in adults at risk.[142] It concludes that the current evidence is insufficient to recommend STI counseling in nonsexually active adults who are not at increased risk for STIs. These recommendations were based on the USPSTF 2008 recommendation statement.

Abbreviations: HIV = human immunodeficiency virus; STI = sexually transmitted infection; USPSTF = U.S. Preventive Services Task Force.

Table 2. Design and Baseline Population Characteristics of Included Studies Targeting Adolescents

Author, year Quality	Setting	Risk	N rand	Intervention Description	Control Description	Age Range (mean, y)	% Female	% Race/ Ethnicity	Currently Sexually Active	STI History
Low-intensity (<30 min)										
Boekeloo, 1999[63,143] Fair	Washington DC, primary care	Low/mix	219	One 15-min audiotape and individual discussion with primary care provider during general health exam	Usual care	12-15 (NR)	50	Black: 63.7 Hispanic: 3.2 White: 18.6 Other: 13.5	Past 3 mo: 21.4%	Treated for STI: 5.9%
Moderate-intensity (30 to 120 min)										
Guilamo-Ramos, 2011[65] Fair	New York, NY, primary care	Low/mix	264	One 30-min individual session with social worker, primary care physician provided brief message, two booster calls with social worker for the mother	Usual care	11-14 (12.9)	52.3	Parent's race/ ethnicity: Black: 15.5 Hispanic: 84.5	6.4%	NR
Danielson, 1990[66] Fair	Portland, OR and Vancouver, WA, HMO	Low/mix	1195	One 1-hr individual counseling session with study health care provider plus slide/ video presentation	No intervention	15-18 (NR)	0	Black: <5 Asian/PI: <4	Past 12 mo: 37%	NR
Kershaw, 2009[59] Fair	Atlanta, GA and New Haven, CT, primary care	Increased	513 (sub-group)	Ten 2-hr prenatal group sessions with midwife or obstetrician, HIV prevention discussion in three sessions (120 min total)	CG1: Attention control (10 2-hr prenatal group sessions with midwife or obstetrician) CG2: Usual prenatal care	14-19 (NR)	100	Black: 80* Hispanic: 13* White: 6* Other: 1*	NR	Lifetime STI: "more than half"*
Kamb (mod IG) 1998[58,144-147] Fair	5 US cities, STI clinic	Increased	508 (sub-group)	IG2: Two 20-min individual counseling sessions with counselor, based on CDC guidelines	CG1: Minimal intervention (two 5-min didactic sessions with physician) CG2: same as CG1, but fewer followup assessments	14-19 (NR)	43*	Black: 59* Hispanic: 19* White: 16* Other: 6*	NR (mean number of sex! partners in past 3 mo, 2.3)	BL STI: 32%*
High-intensity (>120 min)										
Jemmott, 2005[67] Fair	Philadelphia, PA, primary care	Increased	682	IG1: One 4-hr information-based group session with a facilitator IG2: One 4-hr skills-based group session with a facilitator	Attention control (one 4-hr group health promotion session)	12-19 (15.5)	100	Black: 67.9 Hispanic: 32.1	Past 3 mo: 87.1%	BL STI: 21.6%

Table 2. Design and Baseline Population Characteristics of Included Studies Targeting Adolescents

Author, year Quality	Setting	Risk	N rand	Intervention Description	Control Description	Age Range (mean, y)	% Female	% Race/ Ethnicity	Currently Sexually Active	STI History
DiClemente, 2004[68,148-153] Good	Birmingham, AL, primary care	Increased	522	Four 4-hr HIV prevention group sessions with health and peer educators	Attention control (four 4-hr health promotion group sessions)	14-18 (16)	100	Black: 100	Past 6 mo: 100%	BL STI: G: 5.2% C: 17.4% T: 12.6%
Kamb (high IG) 1998[58,144-147] Fair	5 US cities, STI clinic	Increased	512 (sub-group)	IG1: Four 20- to 60-min individual counseling sessions with counselor	CG1: Minimal intervention (two 5-min didactic sessions with physician) CG2: same as CG1, but fewer followup assessments	14-19 (NR)	43*	Black: 59* Hispanic: 19* White: 16* Other: 6*	NR (mean number of sex partners in past 3 mo, 2.3)	BL STI: 32%*
Champion, 2012[69] Fair	Southwestern US, research clinic	Prior STI	559	Three clinical exams and interviews, two motivational workshop sessions, and weekly (3 to 5) support group sessions, plus individual counseling initiated by participants, all with nurse practitioner	Minimal intervention (one session of clinical counseling surrounding STI treatment [time NR] with nurse practitioner)	NR (16.5)	100	Black: 16.4 Hispanic: 83.6	NR (mean age at first intercourse, 13.8 y)	Lifetime STI: 100% (of analyzed sample)
Shain, 1999[57,154-156] Fair	San Antonio, TX, research clinic	Prior STI	148 (sub-group)	Three 3- to 4-hr group cognitive behavioral counseling sessions with facilitator	Minimal intervention (one 15-min standardized individual counseling session per CDC guidelines with nurse clinician)	14-18 (NR)	100	Black: 32 Hispanic: 68	NR (age at first intercourse <15 y, 40.5%)	BL STI: 100%

*Data for entire study population, which included adults and adolescents.

Abbreviations: BL = baseline; C = chlamydia; CDC = Centers for Disease Control and Prevention; CG = control group; G = gonorrhea; HMO = health maintenance organization; HIV = human immunodeficiency virus; IG = intervention group; NR = not reported; rand = randomized; STI = sexually transmitted infection; T = trichomoniasis.

Table 3. Design and Baseline Population Characteristics of Included Studies Targeting Adults

Author, year Quality	Setting	Risk	N rand	Intervention Description	Control Description	Age Range (mean, y)	% Female	% Race/Ethnicity	Sexual History at BL	STI History
Low-intensity (<30 min)										
Proude, 2004[76] Fair	Australia, primary care	General	312	One brief individual session with primary care provider (family physician)	Attention control (tobacco screening and counseling)	18-25 (NR)	71	NR	≥1 sex partners: 78%	NR
Scholes, 2003[83] Fair	WA and NC, primary care	General	1210	Two tailored mailings	Usual care	18-25 (21)	100	Black: 19 White: 69 Other: 12	≥2 sex partners in past 12 mo: 56.5%	Lifetime STI: 27%
Carey (low IG), 2010[84,157,158] Fair	Syracuse, NY, STI clinic	Increased	496	IG1: One 15-min motivational interview with clinic nurse	Minimal intervention (one 15-min educational intervention with clinic nurse)	≥18 (29.2)	46.4	Black: 63.9 Hispanic: 8.7 White: 24.3 Other: 11.9	Mean number of sex partners in past 3 mo: 2.8	BL STI: 18.1%
Peipert, 2008[72,159] Fair	Providence, RI, primary care and Planned Parenthood	Increased	542	Three sessions of tailored computer-based intervention	Minimal intervention (one computer session of standardized contraceptive and STI prevention information [time NR])	13-35 (22)	100	Black: 26 Hispanic: 17 White: 45 Other: 12	≥2 sex partners in past 30 days: 15%	Lifetime STI: 47%
Warner, 2008[78] Good	Denver, CO, Long Beach, CA, and San Francisco, CA, STI clinic	Increased	40,282	One 23-min video on STI/HIV risk and prevention in clinic waiting room	Usual care	NR (NR)	30	Black: 18.5 Hispanic: 25.0 White: 46 Other: 11.0	Men who have sex with men: 31%	BL STI: 15.5%
Jemmott (low IG), 2007[79,160] Good	Newark, NJ, primary care	Increased	322	IG3: One 20-min individual skill intervention with nurses IG4: One 20-min individual information session with nurses	Attention control (general health promotion with nurses)	18-45 (27.2)	100	Black: 100	Mean number of sex partners in past 3 mo: 1.2	BL STI: 20.3%
Marrazzo, 2011[74,161,162] Fair	Seattle, WA, research clinic	Prior STI	89	One education session and motivational interviewing with study staff	Attention control (education session on Pap smears with study staff)	16-30 (25.4)	100	Black: 7.9	>1 female sex partner: 24.7%	Current BV: 100%
Cortes-Bordoy, 2010[86] Fair	Spain, gynecology clinic	Prior STI	211	One counseling session with participant's gynecologist with educational leaflet	Usual care	18-56 (30.2)	100	NR	Mean number of sex partners in past 12 mo: 2.7	Lifetime STI: 100%

Table 3. Design and Baseline Population Characteristics of Included Studies Targeting Adults

Author, year Quality	Setting	Risk	N rand	Intervention Description	Control Description	Age Range (mean, y)	% Female	% Race/ Ethnicity	Sexual History at BL	STI History
Moderate-intensity (30 to 120 min)										
Petersen, 2007[70] Fair	Chapel Hill, NC, primary care	General	764	Two individual STI risk reduction sessions with health educator	Attention control (one preventive health care individual session with health educator)	16-44 (NR)	100	Black: 27￼ White: 62￼ Other: 10	Sexual intercourse in last 30 days: 70%	NR
Wenger, 1992[77] Fair	Los Angeles, CA, primary care	General	435	IG1: One 1-hr HIV/AIDS group education session with study physician IG2: One 1-hr HIV/AIDS group education session with study physician plus HIV testing	No intervention	≥18 (23)	72	Black: 8￼ Hispanic: 13￼ White: 61￼ Asian: 15	Mean number of sex partners in past 30 days: 0.8	Lifetime STI: 23%
Metsch, 2013[90] Good	7 states and Washington, DC, STI clinics	Increased	5012	IG: One HIV testing and risk reduction counseling session with counselor (estimated median of 32 min total)	HIV testing, brief information about HIV according to CDC	≥18 (NR)	34	Black: 41.9￼ Hispanic: 15.3￼ White: 31.8￼ Other: 11.1	Predicted mean number of partners in past 6 mo: 4.65	BL STI: 43.3%
Berenson (mod IG), 2012[71] Fair	Southeast TX, reproductive health clinic	Increased	771	IG1: One 45-min individual contraception and STI counseling with research assistants	Usual care	16-24 (19.9)	100	Black: 18.6￼ Hispanic: 54.2￼ White: 24.8￼ Other: 2.3	Mean number of sex partners in past 12 mo: 1.6	LifetimeSTI: 26.1%
Neumann, 2011[80] Fair	Harlem, NY, and Puerto Rico, STI clinics	Increased	3365	One group session including video and group discussion with facilitator, plus free condoms	Usual care plus free condoms	18-71 (29.3)	51.5	Black: 40.1￼ Hispanic: 50.9￼ White: 0.8￼ Other: 8.2	Same-gender sex: 7.9%	BL STI: 22.2%
Kershaw, 2009[59] Fair	Atlanta, GA, and New Haven, CT, primary care	Increased	1047	Ten 2-hr prenatal group sessions with midwife or obstetrician, HIV prevention discussion in three sessions (120 min total)	CG1: Attention control (10 2-hr prenatal group sessions with midwife or obstetrician) CG2: Usual prenatal care	14-25 (20.4)	100	Black: 80￼ Hispanic: 13￼ White: 6￼ Other: 1	NR	Lifetime STI: "more than half"

Table 3. Design and Baseline Population Characteristics of Included Studies Targeting Adults

Author, year Quality	Setting	Risk	N rand	Intervention Description	Control Description	Age Range (mean, y)	% Female	% Race/ Ethnicity	Sexual History at BL	STI History
Kamb (mod IG), 1998[58,144-147] Fair	5 US cities, STI clinic	Increased	2,890	IG2: Two 20-min individual counseling sessions with counselor, based on CDC guidelines	CG1: Minimal intervention (two 5-min didactic sessions with physician) CG2: same as CG1, but fewer followup assessments	≥14 (25)	43	Black: 59 Hispanic: 19 White: 16 Other: 6	Mean number of sex partners in past 3 mo: 2.3	BL STI: 32%
Crosby, 2009[87] Fair	Southern US, STI clinic	Prior STI	266	One 45- to 50-min peer counseling session with lay health advisors	Minimal intervention ("few minutes" of messaging based on CDC guidelines with nurse, plus 12 free condoms)	18-29 (23.2)	0	Black: 100	Mean number of sex partners in past 3 mo: 3	BL STI: 26%
High-intensity (>120 min)										
Wingood, 2013[89] Good	Atlanta, GA, HMO	Increased	848	Two 4-hr group HIV intervention with health educators	Attention control (nutrition health promotion)	18-29 (22.0)	100	Black: 100	Multiple sex partners in last 6 mo: 36.8%	BL STI: 17%
Berenson (high IG), 2012[71] Fair	Southeast TX, reproductive health clinic	Increased	772	IG2: One 45-min individual contraception and STI counseling with research assistants, 6 to 10 phone calls on correct oral contraceptive and condom use	Usual care	16-24 (19.9)	100	Black: 18.6 Hispanic: 54.2 White: 24.8 Other: 2.3	Mean number of sex partners in past 12 mo: 1.6	Lifetime: 26.1%
Cianelli, 2012[75] Fair	Chile, primary care	Increased	496	Six 2-hr HIV/AIDS prevention group sessions with health educator	Waitlist control	18-49 (32.5)	100	Chilean: 100	NR	NR

Table 3. Design and Baseline Population Characteristics of Included Studies Targeting Adults

Author, year Quality	Setting	Risk	N rand	Intervention Description	Control Description	Age Range (mean, y)	% Female	% Race/ Ethnicity	Sexual History at BL	STI History
Carey (high IG), 2010[84,157,158] Fair	Syracuse, NY, STI clinic	Increased	1235	IG2: 15-min motivational interview plus one 4-hr informational didactic workshop with facilitators IG3: 15-min motivational interview plus one 4-hr information, motivation, and skills workshop with facilitators IG4: CG plus one 4-hr informational workshop with facilitators IG5: CG plus one 4-hr information, motivation, and skills workshop with facilitators	Minimal intervention (one 15-min educational intervention with clinic nurse)	≥18 (29.2)	46.4	Black: 63.9 Hispanic: 8.7 White: 24.3 Other: 11.9	Mean number of sex partners in past 3 mo: 2.8	BL STI: 18.1%
Berkman, 2007[82] Good	New York, NY, psychiatric clinic	Increased	149	Thirteen 1-hr group sessions on HIV risk reduction (Enhanced-SexG) with a substance abuse and/or mental health counselor	Minimal intervention (one HIV presentation that emphasized condom use [time NRJ)/attention control [12 money management sessions])	18-59 (38.6)	0	Black: 54 Hispanic: 28 White: 11 Other: 7	Mean vaginal intercourse with casual partner in past 6 mo: 0.4	NR
Jemmott (high IG), 2007[79,160] Good	Newark, NJ, primary care	Increased	323	IG1: One 3-hr group skills intervention with nurses IG2: One 3-hr group information session with nurses	Attention control (general health promotion with nurses)	18-45 (27.2)	100	Black: 100	Mean number of sex partners in past 3 mo: 1.2	BL STI: 20.3%
Carey, 2004[64] Fair	Syracuse, NY, psychiatric clinic	Increased	408	Ten HIV risk reduction group sessions with facilitators	CG1: Attention control (10 substance abuse group sessions with facilitators) CG2: Usual care	≥18 (36.5)	54	Black: 21 White: 67 Other: 12	Mean number of sex partners in past 3 mo: 1	Lifetime STI: 38%
Ehrhardt, 2002[81,105,163-166] Good	Brooklyn, NY, Planned Parenthood	Increased	360	Eight 2-hr HIV/STI prevention group sessions with facilitators	Minimal intervention (risk assessment only)	18-30 (22.3)	100	Black: 72.5 Hispanic: 16.9 White/other: 10.6	≥2 current male partners: 23.4%	Past 3 mo STI: 16.9%

Behavioral Counseling to Prevent STIs

Kaiser Permanente Research Affiliates EPC

Table 3. Design and Baseline Population Characteristics of Included Studies Targeting Adults

Author, year Quality	Setting	Risk	N rand	Intervention Description	Control Description	Age Range (mean, y)	% Female	% Race/ Ethnicity	Sexual History at BL	STI History
Kamb (high IG) 1998[58,144-147] Fair	5 US cities, STI clinic	Increased	2,881	IG1: Four 20- to 60-min individual counseling sessions with counselor	CG1: Minimal intervention (two 5-min didactic sessions with physician) CG2: same as CG1, but fewer followup assessments	≥14 (25)	43	Black: 59 Hispanic: 19 White: 16 Other: 6	Mean number of sex partners in past 3 mo: 2.3	BL STI: 32%
Marion, 2009[85] Fair	Chicago, IL, primary care	Prior STI	342	Four individual counseling sessions with nurse practitioner and 4 peer-led group classes with a peer educator	Minimal intervention (one 10- to 20-min standardized STI presentation plus STI test and referral to treatment)	≥18 (38.1)	100	Black: 100	Mean number of lifetime sex partners: 26.3	BL STI: 75%
Shain, 2004[73,167] Fair	San Antonio, TX, STI clinic	Prior STI	775	IG1: One 15- to 20-min individual and three 3-hr group cognitive behavioral counseling sessions with facilitator IG2: IG1, plus 5 optional support group sessions	Minimal intervention (one 15- to 20-min STI individual counseling session)	14-43 (21.0)	100	Black: 23.2 Hispanic: 76.8	>1 sex partner in past 3 mo: 25.7%	BL STI: 100%
Shain, 1999[57,154-156] Fair	San Antonio, TX, research clinic	Prior STI	617	Three 3- to 4-hr group cognitive behavioral counseling sessions with facilitator	Minimal intervention (one 15-min standardized individual counseling session per CDC guidelines with nurse clinician)	14-45 (21.6)	100	Black: 31 Hispanic: 69	Mean number of sex partners in last 3 mo: 1.5	BL STI: 100%
Boyer, 1997[88] Fair	San Francisco, CA, STI clinic	Prior STI	393	Four 1-hr individual STI counseling sessions with counselor	Minimal intervention (one 15-min risk reduction individual counseling session with counselor)	18-35 (NR)	32.8	Black: 45.8 Hispanic: 14.5 White: 29.3 Other: 10.2	NR	Lifetime STI: 61.8%

Abbreviations: BL = baseline; CDC = Centers for Disease Control and Prevention; CG = control group; HMO = health maintenance organization; HIV = human immunodeficiency virus; IG = intervention group; NR = not reported; rand = randomized; STI = sexually transmitted infection.

Table 4. Summary of Included Studies—Adolescents

Author, year Quality	Setting	N rand	Population	STI history	Followup Time Points (m)	STI Outcomes	Unprotected Intercourse/ Condom Use	Other Sexual Behavior Outcomes	Other Positive Outcomes
Low-intensity (<30 min)									
Boekeloo, 1999[63,143] Fair	Washington, DC, primary care	219	Adolescents ages 12 to 15 y	Treated for STI: 5.9%	3, 9	↔†	↑↔	↑↔	↔
Moderate-intensity (30 to 120 min)									
Guilamo-Ramos, 2011[65] Fair	New York, NY, primary care	264	African American and Latino adolescents ages 11 to 14 y	NR	9			↑	
Danielson, 1990[66] Fair	Portland, OR and Vancouver, WA, HMO	1195	Adolescent boys ages 15 to 18 y	NR	12		↔		↑
Kershaw, 2009[59] Fair	Atlanta, GA, and New Haven, CT, primary care	513 (subgroup)	Pregnant adolescents age <20 y (NR)	Lifetime STI: "more than half"	3rd trimester, 6, 12	↔			
Kamb (mod IG), 1998[58,144-147] Fair	5 US cities, STI clinic	508 (subgroup)	Sexually active adolescents ages 14 to 19 y	BL STI: 32%*	3, 6, 9, 12	↑			
High-intensity (>120 min)									
Jemmott, 2005[67] Good	Philadelphia, PA, primary care	682	Sexually active African American or Latino adolescent girls ages 12 to 19 y	BL STI: 21.6%	3, 6, 12	↑↔	↑↔	↑↔	
DiClemente, 2004[68,148-153] Good	Birmingham, AL, primary care	522	Sexually active African American adolescent girls ages 14 to 18 y	BL STI: G: 5.2% C: 17.4% T: 12.6%	6, 12	↑↔	↑	↔	↑↔
Kamb (high IG), 1998[58,144-147] Fair	5 US cities, STI clinic	512 (subgroup)	Sexually active adolescents ages 14 to 19 y	BL STI: 32%*	3, 6, 9, 12	↑			
Champion, 2012[69] Fair	Southwestern US, research clinic	559	Ethnic minority adolescent girls with STI or abuse	Lifetime STI: 100% (of analyzed sample)	6, 12	↑			
Shain, 1999[57] Fair	San Antonio, TX, research clinic	148 (subgroup)	Mexican American and African American adolescent girls ages 14 to 18 y with a nonviral STI	BL STI: 100%	6, 12	↑	↔	↑↔	

*Data for entire study population, which included adults and adolescents.
†Self-reported (only or in part) STI outcome.
↑ Results consistently show a benefit of treatment.
↔ Results consistently show no differences between groups.
↑↔ Results are mixed; benefit seen for some outcomes or followups, but not all.

Abbreviations: BL = baseline; C = chlamydia; CG = control group; CI = confidence interval; G = gonorrhea; HIV = human immunodeficiency virus; high= high intensity; IG = intervention group; mod = moderate intensity; NR = not reported; rand = randomized; STI = sexually transmitted infection; T = trichomoniasis.

Behavioral Counseling to Prevent STIs

Kaiser Permanente Research Affiliates EPC

Table 5. Summary of Included Studies—Adults

Author, year Quality	Country, Setting	Risk	N rand	Population (mean age, y)	STI History	Followup Time Points (m)	STI Outcomes	Unprotected Intercourse/ Condom Use	Other Sexual Behavior Outcomes	Other Positive Outcomes	Other Harms
Low-intensity (<30 min)											
Proude, 2004[76] Fair	Australia, primary care	General	312	Adults ages 18 to 25 y	NR	3		↔			
Scholes, 2003[83] Fair	WA and NC, primary care	General	1210	Sexually active nonmonogamous women ages 18 to 24 y	Lifetime STI: 27%	6	↔‖	↑↔			
Carey (low IG), 2010[84,157,158] Fair	Syracuse, NY, STI clinic	Increased	496	Adults age ≥18 y with high-risk behavior in past 3 mo	BL STI: 18.1%	3, 6, 12	↔	↔	↔		↕
Peipert, 2008[159] Fair	Providence, RI, primary care and Planned Parenthood	Increased	542	Women ages 13 to 35 y at high risk for STI or unplanned pregnancy due to age, behavior, history of STI, or pregnancy	Lifetime STI: 47%	24	↔	↔		↕	
Warner, 2008[78] Good	Denver, CO, Long Beach, CA, and San Francisco, CA, STI clinic	Increased	40,282	All patients	BL STI: 15.5%	14.8	↑				
Jemmott (low IG), 2007[79,160] Good	Newark, NJ, primary care	Increased	322	African American women ages 18 to 45 y	BL STI: 20.3%	6, 12	↑↔*	↑↔*			
Marrazzo, 2011[74,161,162] Fair	Seattle, WA, research clinic	Prior STI	89	Women ages 16 to 30 y with bacterial vaginosis who have sex with women	Current BV: 100%	3, 6, 9, 12	↔				
Cortes-Bordoy, 2010[86] Fair	Spain, gynecology clinic	Prior STI	211	Women age ≥18 y with vulvoperineal warts	Lifetime STI: 100%	3, 6, 9, 12		↔	↑	↕	
Moderate-intensity (30 to 120 min)											
Petersen, 2007[70] Fair	Chapel Hill, NC, primary care	General	764	Women ages 16 to 44 y at risk for unintended pregnancy (no IUD or sterilization)	NR	12	↔	↔		↕	
Wenger, 1992[77] Fair	Los Angeles, CA, primary care	General	435	University students age ≥18 y	Lifetime STI: 23%	6		↔	↕		
Metsch, 2013[90] Good	7 states and Washington, DC, STI clinics	Increased	5012	Adults age ≥18 y seeking services at an STI clinic	BL STI: 43.3%	6	↔	↔	↑↔		↕

Table 5. Summary of Included Studies—Adults

Author, year Quality	Country, Setting	Risk	N rand	Population (mean age, y)	STI History	Followup Time Points (m)	STI Outcomes	Unprotected Intercourse/ Condom Use	Other Sexual Behavior Outcomes	Other Positive Outcomes	Other Harms
Berenson (mod IG), 2012[71] Fair	Southeast TX, reproductive health clinic	Increased	771	Sexually active women ages 16 to 24 y	Lifetime STI: 26.1%	3, 6	↔‖	↔		↔	
Neumann, 2011[80] Fair	Harlem, NY, and Puerto Rico, STI clinics	Increased	3365	Adults age ≥18 y, 99% racial/ethnic minority	BL STI: 22.2%	22	↑				
Kershaw, 2009[59] Fair	Atlanta, GA, and New Haven, CT, primary care	Increased	1047	Pregnant women age <25 y	Lifetime STI: "more than half"	3rd tri, 6, 12	↔	↑↔		↑↔	
Kamb (mod IG), 1998[58,144-147] Fair	5 US cities, STI clinic	Increased	4320	Adults and adolescents age ≥14 y	BL STI: 32%	3, 6, 9, 12	↔§	↑↔	↑↔		
Crosby, 2009[87] Fair	Southern US, STI clinic	Prior STI	266	African American men ages 18 to 29 y with newly diagnosed STI and recent experience with condoms	BL STI: 100%	3, 6	↑	↑	↑		
High-intensity (>120 min)											
Wingood, 2013[89] Good	Atlanta, GA, HMO	Increased	848	Sexually active African American women ages 18 to 29 y	BL STI: 17%	6, 12	↑				
Berenson (high IG), 2012[71] Fair	Southeast TX, reproductive health clinic	Increased	772	Sexually active women ages 16 to 24 y	Lifetime STI: 26.1%	3, 6	↔‖	↑		↔	
Cianelli, 2012[75] Fair	Chile, primary care	Increased	496	Chilean women ages 18 to 49 y	NR	3		↔		←	
Carey (high IG), 2010[84,157,158] Fair	Syracuse, NY, STI clinic	Increased	1,235	Adults age ≥18 y with high-risk behavior in past 3 mo	BL STI: 18.1%	3, 6, 12	↔	↔	↔		↔
Berkman, 2007[82] Good	New York, psychiatric clinic	Increased	149	Adult males ages 18 to 59 y with severe mental illness	NR	6, 12		↔	↔		
Jemmott (high IG), 2007[79,160] Fair	Newark, NJ, primary care	Increased	323	African American women ages 18 to 45 y	BL STI: 20.3%	6, 12	↑↔*	↑↔*			
Carey, 2004[64] Fair	Syracuse, NY, psychiatric clinic	Increased	408	Adults age ≥18 y with a mood or thought disorder and alcohol or drug use in past year	Lifetime STI: 38%	3, 6	↑‖	←	↑↔		

Table 5. Summary of Included Studies—Adults

Author, year Quality	Country, Setting	Risk	N rand	Population (mean age, y)	STI History	Followup Time Points (m)	STI Outcomes	Unprotected Intercourse/Condom Use	Other Sexual Behavior Outcomes	Other Positive Outcomes	Other Harms
Ehrhardt, 2002[81,105,163-166] Good	Brooklyn, NY, Planned Parenthood	Increased	360	Women ages 18 to 30 y	Past 3-mo STI: 16.9%	6, 12		↑↔	↑↔	↔	
Kamb (high IG), 1998[58,144-147] Fair	5 US cities, STI clinic	Increased	4311	Adults and adolescents age ≥14 y	BL STI: 32%	3, 6, 9, 12	↔§	↑↔	↑↔		
Marion, 2009[85] Fair	Chicago, IL, primary care	Prior STI	342	Low-income African American women age ≥18 y with ≥2 STIs in the past year	BL STI: 75%	3	↔	↑	↑		↔
Shain, 2004[73,167] Fair	San Antonio, TX, STI clinic	Prior STI	775	Mexican American and African American women ages 15 to 45 y with 1 of 4 STIs	BL STI: 100%	12, 24	↑	↑	↑		
Shain, 1999[57,154-156] Fair	San Antonio, TX, research clinic	Prior STI	617	Mexican American and African American women ages 14 to 45 y with a nonviral STI	BL STI: 100%	6, 12	↔	↑	↑↔		
Boyer, 1997[88] Fair	San Francisco, CA, STI clinic	Prior STI	393	Heterosexual adults ages 18 to 35 y with previous STI, STI symptoms, or known exposure to STI	Lifetime STI: 61.8%	3, 5, 6	↔	↑↔			

*Data not reported separately for high- and low-intensity interventions; instead reported skills-based approach (IG1, IG3) vs. control, skills-based approach (IG1, IG3) vs. information-based approach (IG2, IG4), and high- (IG1) vs. low-intensity (IG3), among skills-based interventions.
†Mail only.
‡Interactive CD-ROM intervention, length NR.
§STI results among adult subgroup only, not entire study population, which includes adults and adolescents.
||Self-reported (only or in part) STI outcome.
↑ Results consistently show a benefit of treatment.
↔ Results consistently show no differences between groups.
↑↔ Results are mixed; benefit seen for some outcomes or followups, but not all.

Abbreviations: BL = baseline; C = chlamydia; CG = control group; CI = confidence interval; G = gonorrhea; IG = intervention group; HIV = human immunodeficiency virus; high = high intensity; low = low intensity; mod = moderate intensity; NR = not reported; rand = randomized; STI = sexually transmitted infection; T = trichomoniasis.

Table 6. Summary of Evidence

Population	# of Studies, Observations (n)	Design	Major limitations	Consistency	Applicability	Overall quality	Summary of Findings
Key Question 1 (Health Outcomes)							
Adolescents	7 trials, 8 comparisons (n=3407)	RCTs (k=5), subgroup analyses from RCTs (k=3)	Little evidence on effects of counseling in boys, race/ethnicity groups other than African Americans and Latinos, and presexually active adolescents	Consistent	Primarily to African American and Latino girls, particularly in low-income urban settings	Fair	Sexual risk reduction counseling generally reduced the odds of STIs in sexually active adolescents in interventions of high (OR, 0.38 [95% CI, 0.24 to 0.60]; k=5; I^2=65%) and moderate (OR, 0.57 [95% CI, 0.37 to 0.86]; k=2; I^2=0%) intensity; data limited for low-intensity interventions; insufficient data on presexually active teens (k=1 in young adolescents, few events).
Adults	19 trials, 23 comparisons (n=61,909)	RCTs (k=19), subgroup analyses from RCTs (k=4)	Almost no evidence on MSM, little data on general- or low-risk primary care settings, no information on adults age ≥50 y	Moderately inconsistent	Primarily to younger adults at increased risk for STIs	Fair	High-intensity interventions reduced odds of STIs by an average of 30% (OR, 0.70 [95% CI, 0.56 to 0.87]; k=9; I^2=23%); most low- and moderate-intensity interventions were not effective and pooled estimates did not demonstrate a benefit of risk reduction counseling, although some promising approaches were identified.
Key Question 2 (Behavioral Outcomes)							
Adolescents	6 trials (n=3030)	RCTs (k=5), subgroup analyses from RCT (k=1)	Same as KQ1, plus inconsistency in outcomes reported, some outcomes sparsely reported	Inconsistent	Primarily to African American and Latino girls, particularly in low-income urban settings	Fair	3 of 5 trials reporting outcomes related to condom use found group differences in at least one outcome, at one or more followup assessments; however, results were frequently inconsistent within studies. Other sexual outcomes were sparsely reported, but 4 trials found improvements in some other sexual outcome. One study showed a temporary increase in sexual activity in inner-city younger adolescents (but no differences in the longer term), but another found reductions in sexual activity in inner-city younger adolescents.
Adults	21 trials, 25 comparisons (n=19,288)	RCTs (k=21) Subgroup analyses from RCTs (k=3)	Same as KQ1, plus inconsistency in outcomes reported, some outcomes sparsely reported	Inconsistent	Primarily to younger adults at increased risk for STIs	Fair	Most high-intensity trials reported improvements in some behavioral outcome at some time point; pooled analysis showed a 29% increase in percent reporting use of condoms in 4 trials (OR, 1.29 [95% CI, 1.13 to 1.48]; I^2=0%). Results in moderate-intensity interventions were mixed and pooled analyses showed a 21% increase in percent reporting use of condoms in 4 trials (OR, 1.21 [95% CI, 1.00 to 1.46]; I^2=28%); 6 low-intensity trials suggested little to no benefit on behavioral outcomes.

Table 6. Summary of Evidence

Population	# of Studies, Observations (n)	Design	Major limitations	Consistency	Applicability	Overall quality	Summary of Findings
Key Question 3 (Other Positive Outcomes)							
Adolescents	3 trials (n=1936)	RCTs	Sparse data for any single outcome, risk for reporting bias	Inconsistent	Very limited	Fair	3 trials reported pregnancy or birth control use; one found a short-term (6 mo) reduction in pregnancy, but group differences did not hold up at 12 mo.
Adults	6 trials (n=4062)	RCTs	Sparse data for any single outcome, risk for reporting bias	Pregnancy outcome consistent, NA for other outcomes	Sexually active women	Fair	4 trials reported no differences in pregnancy, but one increased use of dual contraceptive method use (condom + other) in the intervention group; single trials each reported greater reduction in depression in intervention participants and no differences in intimate partner violence.
Key Question 4 (Harms)							
Adolescents	0 trials	NA	No data	NA	NA	NA	No trials reported on harms; there was no paradoxical increases in STI rate or condom use; no consistent increase in sexual activity.
Adults	3 trials (n=6792)	RCTs	Rarely reported, methods of ascertainment not reported	Consistent	Very limited	Fair	2 trials found no harms of counseling; one trial found more nonserious harms (e.g., pain at finger-stick site) related to HIV test among intervention group than control group. 2 trials showed statistically nonsignificant increases in STIs, but with few events overall.

Abbreviations: CI = confidence interval; HIV = human immunodeficiency virus; KQ = key question; NA = not applicable; OR = odds ratio; RCT = randomized, controlled trial; STI = sexually transmitted infection.

Table 7. Estimated Number Needed to Treat to Prevent One STI and Number of Fewer STIs per 1,000 Persons With Sexual Risk Reduction Counseling

Intervention Intensity and Age Group	% STI in CG	NNT to Prevent One STI	Lower 95% CI	Upper 95% CI	# of Fewer STIs per 1,000	Lower 95% CI	Upper 95% CI
High-intensity intervention in adolescents	5	33	27	52	31	38	20
	15	11	9	18	88	110	55
	25	7	6	12	138	176	84
Moderate-intensity intervention in adolescents	5	48	32	149	21	31	7
	15	17	11	55	59	89	19
	25	11	7	37	91	141	28
High-intensity intervention in adults	5	69	47	161	15	22	7
	15	25	17	59	41	61	17
	25	16	11	40	61	93	26

Abbreviations: CG = control group; CI = confidence interval; NNT = number needed to treat; STI = sexually transmitted infection.

Systematic Review Search Strategies

Cochrane Database of Systematic Reviews search strategy

#1 (hiv OR aids OR hepatitis OR herpes* OR warts OR papilloma*):ti or (hpv OR chlamydia* OR gonorrh* OR syphil*):ti or (std OR stds OR sti OR stis OR sexual*):ti in Cochrane Reviews
#2 (promot* OR educat* OR counsel* OR advice):ti or (advise OR behavio* OR prevent* OR control*):ti in Cochrane Reviews
#3 (#1 AND #2), from 2007 to 2012

Database of Abstracts of Reviews of Effects search strategy

1 (hiv OR aids OR hepatitis OR herpes* OR warts OR papilloma* OR hpv OR chlamydia* OR gonorrh* OR syphil* OR std OR stds OR sti OR stis OR sexual*):TI
2 AND
3 (promot* OR educat* OR counsel* OR advice OR advise OR behavio* OR prevent* OR control*):TI IN FROM 2007 TO 2012

PubMed search strategy

#1 hiv[mesh:noexp] OR hiv infections[mesh:noexp] OR Acquired Immunodeficiency Syndrome[mesh:noexp] OR Hepatitis B[mesh:noexp] OR Hepatitis B, Chronic[mesh:noexp] OR Hepatitis C[mesh:noexp] OR Herpes Simplex[mesh:noexp] OR Herpes Genitalis[mesh:noexp] OR Condylomata Acuminata[mesh:noexp] OR Papillomaviridae[mesh] OR Papillomavirus Infections[mesh:noexp] OR Chlamydia Infections[mesh:noexp] OR Chlamydia[mesh:noexp] OR Chlamydia trachomatis[mesh:noexp] OR Gonorrhea[mesh:noexp] OR Syphilis[mesh:noexp] OR Trichomonas Infections[mesh] OR safe sex[mesh:noexp] OR unsafe sex[mesh:noexp] OR sexual behavior[mesh:noexp] OR Sexually Transmitted Diseases[mesh:noexp] OR Sexually Transmitted Diseases, Bacterial[mesh:noexp] OR Sexually Transmitted Diseases, Viral[mesh:noexp]
#2 health promotion[mesh:noexp] OR Health Education[mesh:noexp] OR patient education as topic[mesh:noexp] OR Counseling[mesh:noexp] OR Directive Counseling[mesh:noexp] OR cognitive therapy[mesh:noexp] OR "motivational interviewing"[tiab] OR behavior therapy[mesh:noexp] OR physician's role[mesh:noexp] OR preventive health services[mesh:noexp] OR student health services[mesh:noexp] OR "preventive intervention"[tiab] OR "preventive interventions"[tiab] OR "prevention intervention"[tiab] OR "prevention interventions"[tiab] OR "behavior intervention"[tiab] OR "behavior interventions"[tiab] OR "behavioral intervention"[tiab] OR "behavioral interventions"[tiab] OR "behaviour intervention"[tiab] OR "behavior interventions"[tiab] OR "behavioural intervention"[tiab] OR "behavioural interventions"[tiab]
#3 #1 AND #2
#4 hiv OR aids OR Hepatitis B OR Hepatitis C OR Herpes OR Herpes OR Condylomata Acuminata OR genital warts OR Papilloma* OR Chlamydia OR Gonorrhea OR Syphilis OR Trichomonas OR "safe sex" OR "unsafe sex" OR "Sexually Transmitted" OR std OR stds OR sti OR stis

#5 "health promotion" OR "Health Education" OR "patient education" OR Counsel* OR "motivational interviewing" OR "preventive intervention"[tiab] OR "preventive interventions"[tiab] OR "prevention intervention"[tiab] OR "prevention interventions"[tiab] OR "behavior intervention"[tiab] OR "behavior interventions"[tiab] OR "behavioral intervention"[tiab] OR "behavioral interventions"[tiab] OR "behaviour intervention"[tiab] OR "behavior interventions"[tiab] OR "behavioural intervention"[tiab] OR "behavioural interventions"[tiab]
#6 #4 AND #5 AND (in process[sb] OR publisher[sb] OR pubmednotmedline[sb])
#7 (#3 OR #6) AND systematic[sb] Filters: Publication date from 2007/01/01; English

Key Question Search Strategies

Database: Ovid MEDLINE(R) without Revisions <1996 to October Week 4 2013 >, Ovid MEDLINE(R) Daily Update <November 1, 2013>, Ovid MEDLINE(R) In-Process & Other Non-Indexed Citations <November 1, 2013>
Search Strategy:
----
1   HIV Infections/ ()
2   Acquired Immunodeficiency Syndrome/ ()
3   Hepatitis B/ ()
4   Hepatitis B, Chronic/ ()
5   Hepatitis C/ ()
6   Hepatitis C, Chronic/ ()
7   Herpes Simplex/ ()
8   Herpes Genitalis/ ()
9   Herpes Labialis/ ()
10   Condylomata Acuminata/ ()
11   Warts/ ()
12   Chlamydia Infections/ ()
13   Gonorrhea/ ()
14   Syphilis/ ()
15   Papillomavirus Infections/ ()
16   Human papillomavirus 6/ ()
17   Human papillomavirus 11/ ()
18   Human papillomavirus 16/ ()
19   Human papillomavirus 18/ ()
20   Trichomonas Infections/ ()
21   Trichomonas Vaginitis/ ()
22   Sexually Transmitted Diseases/ ()
23   Sexually Transmitted Diseases, Bacterial/ ()
24   Sexually Transmitted Diseases, Viral/ ()
25   (hiv or hepatitis or herpes or warts or chlamydia or gonorrhea or syphilis).ti,ab. ()
26   (sexually transmitted or std or stds or sti or stis).ti,ab. ()
27   (papilloma$ or hpv or trichomonas).ti,ab. ()
28   condylomata acuminata.ti,ab. ()

29　1 or 2 or 3 or 4 or 5 or 6 or 7 or 8 or 9 or 10 or 11 or 12 or 13 or 14 or 15 or 16 or 17 or 18 or 19 or 20 or 21 or 22 or 23 or 24 or 25 or 26 or 27 or 28 ()

30　health promotion/ ()

31　Health Education/ ()

32　patient education/ ()

33　counseling/ ()

34　directive counseling/ ()

35　cognitive therapy/ ()

36　behavior therapy/ ()

37　physician's role/ ()

38　preventive health services/ ()

39　student health services/ ()

40　teaching materials/ ()

41　counsel$.ti,ab. ()

42　advice.ti,ab. ()

43　advise.ti,ab. ()

44　motivational interview$.ti,ab. ()

45　prevent$ intervention$.ti,ab. ()

46　health promotion.ti,ab. ()

47　health education.ti,ab. ()

48　patient education.ti,ab. ()

49　cognitive therapy.ti,ab. ()

50　behavio$ therapy.ti,ab. ()

51　behavio$ intervention$.ti,ab. ()

52　30 or 31 or 32 or 33 or 34 or 35 or 36 or 37 or 38 or 39 or 40 or 41 or 42 or 43 or 44 or 45 or 46 or 47 or 48 or 49 or 50 or 51 ()

53　29 and 52 ()

54　Safe Sex/ ()

55　Unsafe Sex/ ()

56　Sexual Behavior/ ()

57　safe sex.ti,ab. ()

58　unsafe sex.ti,ab. ()

59　risky sex$.ti,ab. ()

60　54 or 55 or 56 or 57 or 58 or 59 ()

61　52 and 60 ()

62　HIV Infections/pc ()

63　Acquired Immunodeficiency Syndrome/pc ()

64　Hepatitis B/pc ()

65　Hepatitis B, Chronic/pc ()

66　Hepatitis C/pc ()

67　Hepatitis C, Chronic/pc ()

68　Herpes Simplex/pc ()

69　Herpes Genitalis/pc ()

70　Herpes Labialis/pc ()

71　Condylomata Acuminata/pc ()

72　Warts/pc ()

73   Chlamydia Infections/pc ()
74   Gonorrhea/pc ()
75   Syphilis/pc ()
76   Papillomavirus Infections/pc ()
77   Trichomonas Infections/pc ()
78   Trichomonas Vaginitis/pc ()
79   Sexually Transmitted Diseases/pc ()
80   Sexually Transmitted Diseases, Bacterial/pc ()
81   Sexually Transmitted Diseases, Viral/pc ()
82   62 or 63 or 64 or 65 or 66 or 67 or 68 or 69 or 70 or 71 or 72 or 73 or 74 or 75 or 76 or 77 or 78 or 79 or 80 or 81 ()
83   intervention$.ti,ab,hw. ()
84   82 and 83 ()
85   53 or 61 or 84 ()
86   limit 85 to (clinical trial or controlled clinical trial or meta analysis or randomized controlled trial) ()
87   clinical trials as topic/ or controlled clinical trials as topic/ or randomized controlled trials as topic/ ()
88   Meta-Analysis as Topic/ ()
89   (control$ adj3 trial$).ti,ab. ()
90   random$.ti,ab. ()
91   87 or 88 or 89 or 90 ()
92   85 and 91 ()
93   86 or 92 ()
94   limit 93 to english language ()
95   limit 94 to yr="2007 - 2013" ()
96   remove duplicates from 95 ()

PubMed search strategy (searched only for "publisher" unindexed references)

#1   hiv[tiab] OR aids[tiab] OR "Hepatitis B"[tiab] OR "Hepatitis C"[tiab] OR Herpes[tiab] OR warts[tiab] OR "Condylomata Acuminata"[tiab] OR Papilloma*[tiab] OR hpv[tiab] OR Chlamydia[tiab] OR Gonorrhea[tiab] OR Syphilis[tiab] OR Trichomonas[tiab] OR "safe sex"[tiab] OR "unsafe sex"[tiab] OR "Sexually Transmitted"[tiab] OR std[tiab] OR stds[tiab] OR sti[tiab] OR stis[tiab]
#2   "health promotion"[tiab] OR "Health Education"[tiab] OR "patient education"[tiab]
#3   counsel*[tiab]
#4   "cognitive therapy"[tiab] OR cbt[tiab]
#5   behavio*[tiab] AND (therapy[tiab] OR intervention*[tiab])
#6   advice[tiab] or advise[tiab]
#7   (prevention[tiab] OR preventive[tiab]) AND intervention*[tiab]
#8   motivational[tiab] AND interview*[tiab]
#9   #2 OR #3 OR #4 OR #5 OR #6 OR #7 OR #8
#10   #1 AND #9
#11   #10 AND (trial[tiab] OR trials[tiab] OR random*[tiab] OR metaanaly*[tiab] OR "meta analysis"[tiab] OR "meta analyses"[tiab] OR "meta analytic"[tiab] OR systematic[tiab])

#12   #11 AND publisher[sb]
#13   ((#12) AND English[Language]) AND ("2007"[Date - Publication] : "2013"[Date - Publication])

Cochrane Central Register of Controlled Trials

#1   (hiv or aids or "acquired immunodeficiency" or "human immunodeficiency" or hepatitis or herpes*):ti,ab,kw from 2007 to 2013, in Trials
#2   (hpv or papilloma* or warts or condylomata or trichomonas or chlamydia* or gonorrh* or syphil*):ti,ab,kw from 2007 to 2013, in Trials
#3   (std or stds or sti or stis or sexual*):ti,ab,kw from 2007 to 2013, in Trials
#4   ("safe sex" or "unsafe sex"):ti,ab,kw from 2007 to 2013, in Trials
#5   #1 or #2 or #3 or #4 from 2007 to 2013, in Trials
#6   ("health promotion" or "health education" or "patient education"):ti,ab,kw from 2007 to 2013, in Trials
#7   (counsel* or advise or advice):ti,ab,kw from 2007 to 2013, in Trials
#8   (motivational next interview*):ti,ab,kw from 2007 to 2013, in Trials
#9   (prevention next intervention*):ti,ab,kw from 2007 to 2013, in Trials
#10   "cognitive therapy":ti,ab,kw from 2007 to 2013, in Trials
#11   "physician's role":ti,ab,kw from 2007 to 2013, in Trials
#12   "preventive health services":ti,ab,kw from 2007 to 2013, in Trials
#13   "student health services":ti,ab,kw from 2007 to 2013, in Trials
#14   "teaching materials":ti,ab,kw from 2007 to 2013, in Trials
#15   "client education":ti,ab,kw from 2007 to 2013, in Trials
#16   (behavio* next intervention*):ti,ab,kw from 2007 to 2013, in Trials
#17   (behavio* next therapy):ti,ab,kw from 2007 to 2013, in Trials
#18   (behavio* next change*):ti,ab,kw from 2007 to 2013, in Trials
#19   (behavio* next modification*):ti,ab,kw from 2007 to 2013, in Trials
#20   "preventive medicine":ti,ab,kw from 2007 to 2013, in Trials
#21   (health next behavio*):ti,ab,kw from 2007 to 2013, in Trials
#22   intervention*:ti,ab,kw
#23   #21 and #22
#24   #6 or #7 or #8 or #9 or #10 or #11 or #12 or #13 or #14 or #15 or #16 or #17 or #18 or #19 or #20 or #23 from 2007 to 2013, in Trials
#25   #5 and #24 from 2007 to 2013, in Trials

PsycInfo <1806 to October Week 4 2013>
Searches
1   sexually transmitted diseases/ ()
2   Acquired Immune Deficiency Syndrome/ ()
3   Human Immunodeficiency Virus/ ()
4   GONORRHEA/ ()
5   HERPES GENITALIS/ ()
6   HERPES SIMPLEX/ ()
7   AIDS Prevention/ ()
8   SYPHILIS/ ()

9   HEPATITIS/ ()
10   Human Papillomavirus/ ()
11   Sexual Risk Taking/ ()
12   safe sex/ ()
13   Psychosexual Behavior/ ()
14   sexually transmitted.ti,ab,id. ()
15   aids.ti,ab,id. ()
16   hiv.ti,ab,id. ()
17   hepatitis b.ti,ab,id. ()
18   hepatitis c.ti,ab,id. ()
19   herpes.ti,ab,id. ()
20   condylomata acuminata.ti,ab,id. ()
21   warts.ti,ab,id. ()
22   chlamydia.ti,ab,id. ()
23   gonorrhea.ti,ab,id. ()
24   papillomavirus.ti,ab,id. ()
25   hpv.ti,ab,id. ()
26   trichomonas.ti,ab,id. ()
27   syphilis.ti,ab,id. ()
28   1 or 2 or 3 or 4 or 5 or 6 or 7 or 8 or 9 or 10 or 11 or 12 or 13 or 14 or 15 or 16 or 17 or 18 or 19 or 20 or 21 or 22 or 23 or 24 or 25 or 26 or 27 ()
29   Health Education/ ()
30   Health Promotion/ ()
31   Cognitive behavior therapy/ ()
32   Behavior Therapy/ ()
33   Behavior Change/ ()
34   Behavior Modification/ ()
35   Client Education/ ()
36   Counseling/ ()
37   Preventive Medicine/ ()
38   student personnel services/ ()
39   Lifestyle Changes/ ()
40   advice.ti,ab,id. ()
41   advise.ti,ab,id. ()
42   counsel$.ti,ab,id,hw. ()
43   prevention intervention$.ti,ab,id. ()
44   motivational interview$.ti,ab,id. ()
45   behavio$ intervention$.ti,ab,id. ()
46   Health Behavior/ ()
47   46 and intervention$.ti,ab,id. ()
48   health promotion.ti,ab,id. ()
49   health education.ti,ab,id. ()
50   behavio$ therapy.ti,ab,id. ()
51   behavio$ change$.ti,ab,id. ()
52   behavio$ modification$.ti,ab,id. ()
53   client education.ti,ab,id. ()

Appendix A. Detailed Methods

54   29 or 30 or 31 or 32 or 33 or 34 or 35 or 36 or 37 or 38 or 39 or 40 or 41 or 42 or 43 or 44 or 45 or 47 or 48 or 49 or 50 or 51 or 52 or 53 ()
55   28 and 54 ()
56   random$.ti,ab,id,hw. ()
57   controlled trial$.ti,ab,id,hw. ()
58   clinical trial$.ti,ab,id,hw. ()
59   treatment outcome clinical trial.md. ()
60   56 or 57 or 58 or 59 ()
61   55 and 60 ()
62   limit 61 to english language ()
63   limit 62 to yr="2007 - 2014" ()

Appendix A Figure 1. Literature Flow Diagram

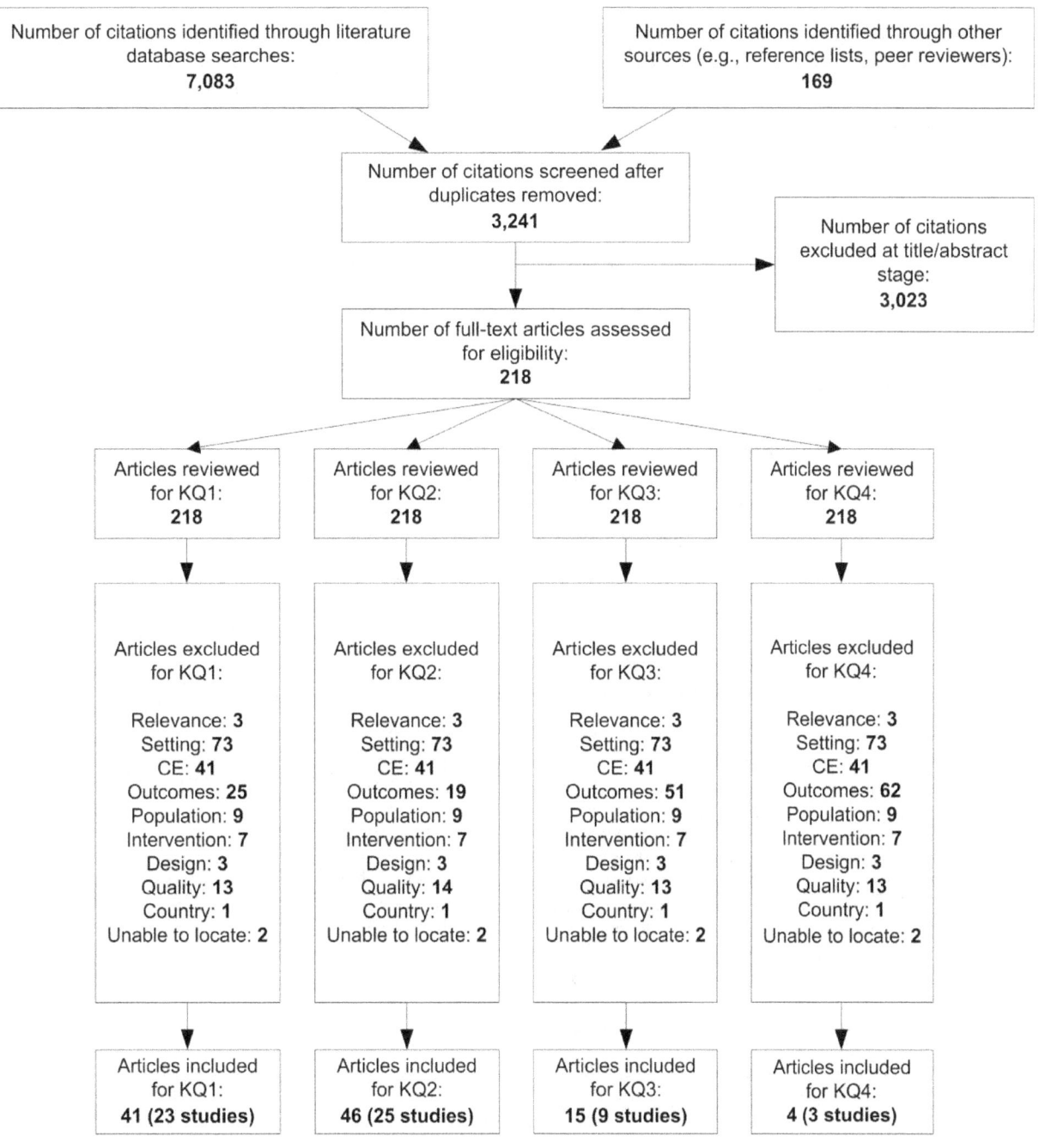

Abbreviations: CE = comparative effectiveness; KQ = key question.

Appendix A Table 1. Inclusion and Exclusion Criteria

Category	Inclusion	Exclusion
Aim	Targeting sexual behavior change to prevent HIV/STIs (may also target additional behaviors)	Only targeting sexual behavior change to prevent unintended pregnancy or another behavior associated with risky sexual behavior (e.g., alcohol misuse, drug abuse)
Condition	An STI is any infection that is transmitted through sexual contact (i.e., oral, vaginal, or anal)[1]	Other methods by which bloodborne STIs can be acquired (e.g., maternal-fetal transmission, blood transfusions, inadvertent needle sticks, sharing needles or injection equipment with a potentially infected person)
Population	• Men and women of all ages, of any sexual orientation, including pregnant women • Sexually active or not	• HIV-positive (>10% of study population) • Current inmates, juvenile offenders, court-involved individuals • Psychiatric inpatients
Interventions	Primary care conducted, feasible,* or referable intervention involving behavioral counseling to prevent or reduce HIV/STIs (i.e., some provision of education, skills training, or guidance on how to change sexual behaviors) delivered alone or in combination with other interventions intended to promote sexual risk reduction or risk avoidance Interventions may include, but are not limited to, individual-, family-, couple-, or group-based counseling (e.g., motivational interviewing, cognitive behavioral counseling), abstinence contracts with provider, virtual- or technology-based interventions (e.g., text messages), HIV counseling and testing, case management, and skills training *Criteria for feasibility: • Whom targeted: individual-level identification of being a patient/in need of intervention • Who delivered: usually involves primary care clinicians (family practice, internal medicine, obstetrics/gynecology, pediatrics, or general practitioners), other physicians, nurses, nurse practitioners, physician assistants, or related clinical staff (dietitians, health educators, mental health practitioners, or other counselors) in some direct or indirect way, or is seen as connected to the health care system by the participant • How delivered: to individuals or in small groups (≤15 patients) • Where delivered: could be delivered anywhere (including via the Web, interactive technology, in the home), as long as linked to a health care provider or system • Components: must not include components that cannot be replicated in most health care settings, including environmental components (media messages, signage), or that intervenes on groups in closed (preexisting) social networks (e.g., worksites, churches) or uses authority figures (e.g., military commanders, workplace supervisors)	• Trials within closed preexisting social networks (e.g., worksite or church programs) • School programs outside school-based health clinics • Social marketing (e.g., media campaigns) • Policy (e.g., state or local public or health policy; health care delivery) • Circumcision to prevent HIV/STIs; circumcision counseling • Biomedical HIV/STI prevention interventions (e.g., prophylactic vaccinations, antiretroviral therapy in high-risk individuals) or counseling to increase use • Promoting HIV/STI testing • Maternal-to-fetal transmission prevention counseling • Sexual abuse prevention • Cash incentives for behavior change (e.g., condom use) • Counseling to increase partner referral or notification only • Contraceptive use • Complementary and alternative medicine (e.g., hypnosis)

Appendix A Table 1. Inclusion and Exclusion Criteria

Category	Inclusion	Exclusion
Comparators	<ul><li>No intervention (e.g., waitlist)</li><li>Usual care</li><li>Minimal intervention (e.g., usual care limited to ≤15 min of information)</li><li>Attention control (e.g., similar in format and intensity, but intervention is on a different content area, such as general sex education, wellness promotion, or nutrition education)</li></ul>	Active intervention (i.e., comparative effectiveness)
Outcomes	**KQ 1: Health outcomes**<ul><li>STI incidence (testing and self-report)</li><li>STI-related morbidity and mortality, including: cancer (e.g., liver, oral, cervical, vulvular, vaginal, anal, penile, Kaposi's sarcoma, non-Hodgkin's lymphoma), reproductive health problems (e.g., pelvic inflammatory disease, ectopic pregnancy, spontaneous abortion, infertility, epididymitis, prostatitis), maternal problems (e.g., preterm delivery, premature rupture of membranes, puerperal sepsis, postpartum infection), infant problems (e.g., stillbirth, low birth weight, ophthalmia neonatorum [caused by gonorrhea, herpes simplex virus, or chlamydia], pneumonia, neonatal sepsis, congenital HIV, congenital syphilis, acute hepatitis, neurologic damage, congenital abnormalities), AIDS, other (e.g., oral lesions, meningitis, neurosyphilis, chronic liver disease, pelvic pain, genitourinary complaint), or death from any of these conditions</li></ul>**KQ 2: Behavioral outcomes**<ul><li>Changes in sexual behavior, including risky behaviors (e.g., multiple [new] partners, high-risk partners, unprotected vaginal or anal intercourse, other contact with bodily fluid, sex while intoxicated with alcohol or other substances, sex in exchange for money or drugs)</li><li>Changes in protective behaviors (e.g., abstinence, mutual monogamy, delayed initiation of intercourse or age of sexual debut, decreased contact with bodily fluids [use of condoms, other barrier methods, chemical barriers, or other changes in sexual behavior])</li><li>Sexual negotiation skills (trial must also report change in risky or protective behavior listed above or a health outcome)</li></ul>**KQ 3: Other positive outcomes**<ul><li>Reduction in unintended pregnancy</li><li>Others based on target populations (e.g., decrease in substance abuse/misuse among current drug users)</li></ul>**KQ 4: Adverse events**<ul><li>Paradoxical increase in STI incidence or risky sexual behaviors or decrease in protective behaviors</li><li>Care avoidance</li><li>Shame, guilt</li><li>Stigma</li></ul>	Self-reported measures of attitude, knowledge, ability, or self-efficacy (e.g., knowledge of HIV/STI risk and transmission, knowledge of protective behaviors, perception of HIV/STI risk in self or partners, regretted intercourse, participation in AIDS-related community activities, perceived powerlessness), sexual negotiation skills, scheduling a health care appointment or discussing its importance with family, intention to use protective barriers, or carrying barrier protection

Appendix A Table 1. Inclusion and Exclusion Criteria

Category	Inclusion	Exclusion
Intervention setting	• Primary care settings (e.g., pediatric, obstetrics/gynecology, internal medicine, family practice, family planning, military, adolescent and school-based health clinics) • Mental health clinics • STI and family planning clinics • Virtual (e.g., online counseling)	• Community/university research laboratories or other nonmedical centers • Correctional facilities • School classrooms • Worksites • Substance abuse treatment facilities or methadone maintenance clinics • Inpatient/residential facilities • Emergency departments
Study design	Randomized, controlled trials and nonrandomized, controlled trials (controlled clinical trials)	Observational studies, comparative effectiveness trials without a control group
Timing of outcome assessment	≥3 months postbaseline	<3 months postbaseline
Publication date (not search date)	Published after 1987 (1988 to present; post-HIV/AIDS era)	Published in or before 1987
Country	Countries with a Human Development Index of "Very High"	Countries with a Human Development Index below "Very High"
Language	English only	Non-English publications
Study quality	Fair or good	Poor (e.g., <60% retention overall)

Appendix A Table 2. Quality Assessment Tool

Design	U.S. Preventive Services Task Force Quality Rating Criteria[56]
Systematic reviews and meta-analyses	• Comprehensiveness of sources considered/search strategy used • Standard appraisal of included studies • Validity of conclusions • Recency and relevance are especially important for systematic reviews
Randomized, controlled trials	• Initial assembly of comparable groups employs adequate randomization, including first concealment and whether potential confounders were distributed equally among groups • Maintenance of comparable groups (includes attrition, crossovers, adherence, contamination) • Important differential loss to followup or overall high loss to followup • Measurements are equal, reliable, and valid (includes masking of outcome assessment) • Clear definition of the interventions • All important outcomes considered

Appendix B. Excluded Studies

Exclusion code key

E1. Study relevance/aim
E2a. Setting: Not one of the specified settings
E2b. Setting: Setting is substance abuse treatment center
E2c. Setting: Not linked to primary care
E3. Comparative effectiveness (control group received active intervention)
E4. No relevant outcomes
E5a. Population: Limited to HIV+ individuals
E5b. Population: Limited to other populations (inmates, juvenile offenders, court-involved, psychiatric inpatients)
E6. Intervention
E7. Study design: Not a randomized or controlled clinical trial
E8a. Study quality: High or differential attrition
E8b. Study quality: Other quality issue
E8c. Study quality: Timing of outcome assessment <3 mo
E9. Non-English language
E10. Non-high HDI country
E11. Published in 1987 or earlier
E12. Not able to locate full text

1. The NIMH Multisite HIV Prevention Trial: reducing HIV sexual risk behavior. The National Institute of Mental Health (NIMH) Multisite HIV Prevention Trial Group. Science 1998;280(5371):1889-94. PMID: 9632382. **KQ1E3, KQ2E3, KQ3E3, KQ4E3.**

2. Social-cognitive theory mediators of behavior change in the National Institute of Mental Health Multisite HIV Prevention Trial. Health Psychol 2001;20(5):369-76. PMID: 11570651. **KQ1E3, KQ2E3, KQ3E3, KQ4E3.**

3. Akers DD. ASSESS: For adolescent risk reduction. In: Card JJ, Benner TA (eds). Model Programs for Adolescent Sexual Health: Evidence-based HIV, STI, and Pregnancy Prevention Interventions. New York, NY: Springer Publishing Company, LLC; 2008. p. 375-82. PMID: None. **KQ4E4.**

4. Alemagno SA, Stephens RC, Stephens P, et al. Brief motivational intervention to reduce HIV risk and to increase HIV testing among offenders under community supervision. J Correct Health Care 2009 Jul;15(3):210-21. PMID: 19477803. **KQ1E8c, KQ2E8c, KQ3E8c, KQ4E8c.**

5. Bangi A, Dolcini MM, Harper GW, et al. Psychosocial outcomes of sexual risk reduction in a brief intervention for urban African American female adolescents. J HIV AIDS Soc Serv 2013 Apr;12(2):146-59. PMID: 24039550. **KQ1E2c, KQ2E2c, KQ3E2c, KQ4E2c.**

6. Barresi P, Husnik M, Camacho M, et al. Recruitment of men who have sex with men for large HIV intervention trials: analysis of the EXPLORE study recruitment effort. AIDS Educ Prev 2010 Feb;22(1):28-36. PMID: 20166785. **KQ1E2a, KQ2E2a, KQ3E2a, KQ4E2a.**

7. Bedoya CA, Mimiaga MJ, Beauchamp G, et al. Predictors of HIV transmission risk behavior and seroconversion among Latino men who have sex with men in Project EXPLORE. AIDS Behav 2012 Apr;16(3):608-17. PMID: 21390540. **KQ1E2a, KQ2E2a, KQ3E2a, KQ4E2a.**

8. Belcher L, Kalichman S, Topping M, et al. A randomized trial of a brief HIV risk reduction counseling intervention for women. J Consult Clin Psychol 1998;66(5):856-61. PMID: 9803706. **KQ1E2c, KQ2E2c, KQ3E2c, KQ4E2c.**

9. Benner TA. What Could You Do? Interactive video intervention to reduce adolescent females' STI risk. In: Card JJ, Benner TA (eds). Model Program for Adolescent Sexual Health: Evidence-based HIV, STI and Pregnancy Prevention Interventions. New York, NY: Springer Publishing Company, LLC; 2008. p. 227-34. PMID: None. **KQ1E3, KQ2E3, KQ3E3, KQ4E3.**

10. Benner TA. SiHLE: Health workshops for young black women. In: Card JJ, Benner TA (eds). Model Programs for Adolescent Sexual Health: Evidence-based HIV, STI and Pregnancy Prevention Interventions. New York, NY: 2008. p. 253-60. PMID: None. **KQ4E4.**

Appendix B. Excluded Studies

11. Benner TA. FOCUS: Preventing sexually transmitted infections and unwanted pregnancies among young women. In: Card JJ, Benner TA (eds). Model Programs for Adolescent Sexual Health: Evidence-based HIV, STI and Pregnancy Prevention Interventions. New York, NY: Springer Publishing Company, LLC; 2008. p. 217-26. PMID: None. **KQ1E2a, KQ2E2a, KQ3E2a, KQ4E2a.**

12. Berenson AB, Rahman M. A randomized controlled study of two educational interventions on adherence with oral contraceptives and condoms. Contraception 2012 Dec;86(6):716-24. PMID: 22840278. **KQ4E4.**

13. Berenson AB. A study of two interventions to increase adherence with oral contraceptives and condom use among adolescents and young adults. Dissertation Abstracts International: Section B: The Sciences and Engineering 2013;73(11-B) PMID: None. **KQ1E12, KQ2E12, KQ3E12, KQ4E12.**

14. Berkman A. Reducing sexual risk behaviors of men with severe mental illness. J Consult Clin Psychol 2006;57(3):417. PMID: 16525006. **KQ1E7, KQ2E7, KQ3E7, KQ4E7.**

15. Berkman A, Cerwonka E, Sohler N, et al. A randomized trial of a brief HIV risk reduction intervention for men with severe mental illness. J Consult Clin Psychol 2006 Mar;57(3):407-9. PMID: 16525002. **KQ1E3, KQ2E3, KQ3E3, KQ4E3.**

16. Berkman A, Pilowsky DJ, Zybert PA, et al. HIV prevention with severely mentally ill men: a randomised controlled trial. AIDS Care 2007 May;19(5):579-88. PMID: 17505917. **KQ1E4, KQ3E4, KQ4E4.**

17. Boekeloo BO, Schamus LA, Simmens SJ, et al. A STD/HIV prevention trial among adolescents in managed care. Pediatrics 1999 Jan;103(1):107-15. PMID: 9917447. **KQ4E4.**

18. Bolu OO, Lindsey C, Kamb ML, et al. Is HIV/sexually transmitted disease prevention counseling effective among vulnerable populations?: a subset analysis of data collected for a randomized, controlled trial evaluating counseling efficacy (Project RESPECT). Sex Transm Dis 2004 Aug;31(8):469-74. PMID: 15273579. **KQ2E4, KQ3E4, KQ4E4.**

19. Bowen AM, Horvath K, Williams ML. A randomized control trial of Internet-delivered HIV prevention targeting rural MSM. Health Educ Res 2007 Feb;22(1):120-7. PMID: 16849391. **KQ1E2c, KQ2E2c, KQ3E2c, KQ4E2c.**

20. Boyer CB, Barrett DC, Peterman TA, et al. Sexually transmitted disease (STD) and HIV risk in heterosexual adults attending a public STD clinic: evaluation of a randomized controlled behavioral risk-reduction intervention trial. AIDS 1997 Mar;11(3):359-67. PMID: 9147428. **KQ3E4, KQ4E4.**

21. Branson BM, Peterman TA, Cannon RO, et al. Group counseling to prevent sexually transmitted disease and HIV: a randomized controlled trial. Sex Transm Dis 1998 Nov;25(10):553-60. **KQ1E3, KQ2E3, KQ3E3, KQ4E3.**

22. Bull S, Pratte K, Whitesell N, et al. Effects of an Internet-based intervention for HIV prevention: the Youthnet trials. AIDS & Behav 2009 Jun;13(3):474-87. PMID: 19037719. **KQ1E3, KQ2E3, KQ3E3, KQ4E3.**

23. Bull SS, Levine DK, Black SR, et al. Social media-delivered sexual health intervention: a cluster randomized controlled trial. Am J Prev Med 2012 Nov;43(5):467-74. PMID: 23079168. **KQ1E2c, KQ2E2c, KQ3E2c, KQ4E2c.**

24. Callahan EJ, Flynn NM, Kuenneth CA, et al. Strategies to reduce HIV risk behavior in HIV primary care clinics: brief provider messages and specialist intervention. AIDS & Behav 2007 Sep;11(5:Suppl):S48-S57. PMID: 17205389. **KQ1E4, KQ2E4, KQ3E4, KQ4E4.**

25. Calsyn DA, Hatch-Maillette M, Tross S, et al. Motivational and skills training HIV/sexually transmitted infection sexual risk reduction groups for men. J Subst Abuse Treat 2009 Sep;37(2):138-50. PMID: 19150206. **KQ1E3, KQ2E3, KQ3E3, KQ4E3.**

26. Calsyn DA, Burlew AK, Hatch-Maillette MA, et al. An HIV prevention intervention for ethnically diverse men in substance abuse treatment: pilot study findings. Am J Public Health 2013 May;103(5):896-902. PMID: 23488494. **KQ1E3, KQ2E3, KQ3E3, KQ4E3.**

Appendix B. Excluded Studies

27. Campbell AN, Tross S, Hu MC, et al. Female condom skill and attitude: results from a NIDA Clinical Trials Network gender-specific HIV risk reduction study. AIDS Educ Prev 2011 Aug;23(4):329-40. PMID: 21861607. **KQ1E2b, KQ2E2b, KQ3E2b, KQ4E2b.**

28. Card JJ, Kuhn T, Solomon J, et al. Translating an effective group-based HIV prevention program to a program delivered primarily by a computer: methods and outcomes. AIDS Educ Prev 2011 Apr;23(2):159-74. PMID: 10.1521/aeap.2011.23.2.159 [doi];10.1521/aeap.2011.23.2.159 [pii]. **KQ1E3, KQ2E3, KQ3E3, KQ4E3.**

29. Carey MP, Carey KB, Maisto SA, et al. Reducing HIV-risk behavior among adults receiving outpatient psychiatric treatment: results from a randomized controlled trial. J Consult Clin Psychol 2004 Apr;72(2):252-68. PMID: 15065959. **KQ3E4, KQ4E4.**

30. Carey MP, Vanable PA, Senn TE, et al. Evaluating a two-step approach to sexual risk reduction in a publicly-funded STI clinic: rationale, design, and baseline data from the Health Improvement Project-Rochester (HIP-R). Contemp Clin Trials 2008 Jul;29(4):569-86. PMID: 18325853. **KQ3E4, KQ4E4.**

31. Carey MP, Senn TE, Vanable PA, et al. Brief and intensive behavioral interventions to promote sexual risk reduction among STD clinic patients: results from a randomized controlled trial. AIDS & Behav 2010 Jun;14(3):504-17. PMID: 19590947. **KQ3E4.**

32. Carpenter KM, Stoner SA, Mikko AN, et al. Efficacy of a web-based intervention to reduce sexual risk in men who have sex with men. AIDS & Behav 2010 Jun;14(3):549-57. PMID: 19499321. **KQ1E2c, KQ2E2c, KQ3E2c, KQ4E2c.**

33. Castor D, Pilowsky DJ, Hadden B, et al. Sexual risk reduction among non-injection drug users: report of a randomized controlled trial. AIDS Care 2010 Jan;22(1):62-70. PMID: 20390482. **KQ1E2c, KQ2E2c, KQ3E2c, KQ4E2c.**

34. Champion JD. Behavioural interventions and abuse: secondary analysis of reinfection in minority women. Int J STD AIDS 2007 Nov;18(11):748-53. PMID: 18005508. **KQ2E4, KQ3E4, KQ4E4.**

35. Champion JD, Collins J. African-and Mexican-American Adolescent women with sti and a history of abuse: Biological outcome of a randomised trial of behavioural intervention. Sex Transm Infect 2011;87(Suppl 1):A266. PMID: None. **KQ1E4, KQ2E4, KQ3E4, KQ4E4.**

36. Champion JD, Collins JL. Comparison of a theory-based (AIDS Risk Reduction Model) cognitive behavioral intervention versus enhanced counseling for abused ethnic minority adolescent women on infection with sexually transmitted infection: results of a randomized controlled trial. Int J Nurs Stud 2012 Feb;49(2):138-50. PMID: 21937041 **KQ2E4, KQ3E4, KQ4E4.**

37. Chawarski MC, Mazlan M, Schottenfeld RS. Behavioral drug and HIV risk reduction counseling with abstinence-contingent take-home buprenorphine: A pilot randomized clinical trial. Drug Alcohol Depend 2007;94(1-3):281-4. PMID: 18164145. **KQ1E2b, KQ2E2b, KQ3E2b, KQ4E2b.**

38. Choi KH, Hoff C, Gregorich SE, et al. The efficacy of female condom skills training in HIV risk reduction among women: a randomized controlled trial. Am J Public Health 2008 Oct;98(10):1841-8. PMID: 18703460. **KQ1E3, KQ2E3, KQ3E3, KQ4E3.**

39. Cianelli R, Ferrer L, Norr KF, et al. Mano a Mano-Mujer: an effective HIV prevention intervention for Chilean women. Health Care Women Int 2012;33(4):321-41. PMID: 22420675. **KQ1E4, KQ4E4.**

40. Cohen DA, Dent C, MacKinnon D, et al. Condom skills education and sexually transmitted disease reinfection. J Sex Res 1991;28(1):139-45. PMID: None. **KQ1E8b, KQ2E8b, KQ3E8b, KQ4E8b.**

41. Collins PY, von UH, Putnins S, et al. Adding the female condom to HIV prevention interventions for women with severe mental illness: a pilot test. Community Ment Health J 2011 Apr;47(2):143-55. PMID: 20336486. **KQ1E5b, KQ2E5b, KQ3E5b, KQ4E5b.**

42. Cortes-Bordoy J, Vidart JA, Coll-Capdevila C, et al. Usefulness of an educational leaflet to modify sexual risk behaviour in women with external genital warts. Eur J Dermatol 2010 May;20(3):339-44. PMID: 20146965. **KQ1E4, KQ3E4, KQ4E4.**

Appendix B. Excluded Studies

43. Cottler LB, Compton WM, Ben AA, et al. Peer-delivered interventions reduce HIV risk behaviors among out-of-treatment drug abusers. Public Health Rep 1998 Jun;113 Suppl 1:31-41. **KQ1E3, KQ2E3, KQ3E3, KQ4E3.**

44. Crosby R, DiClemente RJ, Charnigo R, et al. A brief, clinic-based, safer sex intervention for heterosexual African American men newly diagnosed with an STD: a randomized controlled trial. Am J Public Health 2009 Apr;99(Suppl 1):S96-S103. PMID: 19218185. **KQ3E4, KQ4E4.**

45. Dancy BL, Dancy BL. African American adolescent females: Mother-involved HIV risk-reduction intervention. Journal of HIV/AIDS & Social Services 2009 Jul;8(3):292-307. PMID: 20090855. **KQ1E8b, KQ2E8b, KQ3E8b, KQ4E8b.**

46. Danielson CK, McCauley JL, Jones AM, et al. Feasibility of Delivering Evidence-Based HIV/STI Prevention Programming to a Community Sample of African American Teen Girls Via the Internet. AIDS Education & Prevention 2013 Oct;25(5):394-404. **KQ1E2c, KQ2E2c, KQ3E2c, KQ4E2c.**

47. Danielson R, Marcy S, Plunkett A, et al. Reproductive health counseling for young men: what does it do? Fam Plann Perspect 1990 May;22(3):115-21. PMID: 2379568. **KQ1E4, KQ4E4.**

48. Davey-Rothwell MA, Tobin K, Yang C, et al. Results of a randomized controlled trial of a peer mentor HIV/STI prevention intervention for women over an 18 month follow-up. AIDS & Behav 2011 Nov;15(8):1654-63. PMID: 21468659. **KQ1E6, KQ2E6, KQ3E6, KQ4E6.**

49. Dermen KH, Thomas SN. Randomized controlled trial of brief interventions to reduce college students' drinking and risky sex. Psychol Addict Behav 2011 Dec;25(4):583-94. PMID: 21928866. **KQ1E2a, KQ2E2a, KQ3E2a, KQ4E2a.**

50. Di NJ, Schinke SP. Gender-specific HIV prevention with urban early-adolescent girls: outcomes of the Keepin' It Safe Program. AIDS Educ Prev 2007 Dec;19(6):479-88. PMID: 18190273. **KQ1E2a, KQ2E2a, KQ3E2a, KQ4E2a.**

51. Diallo DD, Moore TW, Ngalame PM, et al. Efficacy of a single-session HIV prevention intervention for black women: a group randomized controlled trial. AIDS & Behav 2010 Jun;14(3):518-29. PMID: 20135214. **KQ1E6, KQ2E6, KQ3E6, KQ4E6.**

52. DiClemente RJ, Wingood GM, Harrington KF, et al. Efficacy of an HIV prevention intervention for African American adolescent girls: a randomized controlled trial. JAMA 2004 Jul 14;292(2):171-9. PMID: 15249566. **KQ4E4.**

53. DiClemente RJ, Wingood GM, Rose ES, et al. Efficacy of sexually transmitted disease/human immunodeficiency virus sexual risk-reduction intervention for african american adolescent females seeking sexual health services: a randomized controlled trial. Arch Pediatr Adolesc Med 2009 Dec;163(12):1112-21. PMID: 19996048. **KQ1E3, KQ2E3, KQ3E3, KQ4E3.**

54. DiClemente RJ, Wingood GM, Rose E, et al. Evaluation of an HIV/STD sexual risk-reduction intervention for pregnant African American adolescents attending a prenatal clinic in an urban public hospital: preliminary evidence of efficacy. J Pediatr Adolesc Gynecol 2010 Feb;23(1):32-8. PMID: 19643646. **KQ1E8a, KQ2E8a, KQ3E8a, KQ4E8a.**

55. DiClemente RJ, Brown JL, Sales JM, et al. Rate of decay in proportion of condom-protected sex acts among adolescents after participation in an HIV risk-reduction intervention. JAIDS 2013 Jun 1;63(Suppl 1):S85-S89. PMID: 23673893. **KQ1E3, KQ2E3, KQ3E3, KQ4E3.**

56. DiIorio C, McCarty F, Resnicow K, et al. REAL men: a group-randomized trial of an HIV prevention intervention for adolescent boys. Am J Public Health 2007 Jun;97(6):1084-9. PMID: 17463382. **KQ1E2a, KQ2E2a, KQ3E2a, KQ4E2a.**

57. Dilley JW, Woods WJ, Sabatino J, et al. Changing sexual behavior among gay male repeat testers for HIV: a randomized, controlled trial of a single-session intervention. J Acquir Immune Defic Syndr 2002 Jun 1;30(2):177-86. **KQ1E8a, KQ2E8a, KQ3E8a, KQ4E8a.**

58. Dilley JW, Woods WJ, Loeb L, et al. Brief cognitive counseling with HIV testing to reduce sexual risk among men who have sex with men: results from a randomized controlled trial using paraprofessional counselors. J Acquir Immune Defic Syndr 2007 Apr 15;44(5):569-77. PMID: 17310937. **KQ1E3, KQ2E3, KQ3E3, KQ4E3.**

59. Dilley JW, Loeb L, Marson K, et al. Sexual compulsiveness and change in unprotected anal intercourse: unexpected results from a randomized controlled HIV counseling intervention study. J Acquir Immune Defic Syndr 2008 May 1;48(1):113-4. PMID: 18438179. **KQ1E3, KQ2E3, KQ3E3, KQ4E3.**

60. Dilley JW, Schwarcz S, Murphy J, et al. Efficacy of personalized cognitive counseling in men of color who have sex with men: secondary data analysis from a controlled intervention trial. AIDS & Behav 2011 Jul;15(5):970-5. PMID: 20680432. **KQ1E3, KQ2E3, KQ3E3, KQ4E3.**

61. Dunn KE, Saulsgiver KA, Patrick ME, et al. Characterizing and improving HIV and hepatitis knowledge among primary prescription opioid abusers. Drug Alcohol Depend 2013 Aug 30 **KQ1E7, KQ2E7, KQ3E7, KQ4E7.**

62. Dworkin SL, Beckford ST, Ehrhardt AA. Sexual scripts of women: a longitudinal analysis of participants in a gender-specific HIV/STD prevention intervention. Arch Sex Behav 2007 Apr;36(2):269-79. PMID: 17186128. **KQ1E4, KQ3E4, KQ4E4.**

63. Eaton LA, Cherry C, Cain D, et al. A novel approach to prevention for at-risk HIV-negative men who have sex with men: creating a teachable moment to promote informed sexual decision-making. Am J Public Health 2011 Mar;101(3):539-45. PMID: 21233441. **KQ1E2a, KQ2E2a, KQ3E2a, KQ4E2a.**

64. Eaton LA. The development and outcomes of an intervention to address serosorting among HIV negative men who have sex with men. Storrs-Mansfield, CT: University of Connecticut; 2010. **KQ1E2a, KQ2E2a, KQ3E2a, KQ4E2a.**

65. Ehrhardt AA, Exner TM, Hoffman S, et al. A gender-specific HIV/STD risk reduction intervention for women in a health care setting: short- and long-term results of a randomized clinical trial. AIDS Care 2002 Apr;14(2):147-61. PMID: 11940275. **KQ1E4, KQ4E4.**

66. El-Bassel N, Witte SS, Gilbert L, et al. The efficacy of a relationship-based HIV/STD prevention program for heterosexual couples. Am J Public Health 2003;93(6):963-9. PMID: 12773363. **KQ1E3, KQ2E3, KQ3E3, KQ4E3.**

67. El-Bassel N, Witte SS, Gilbert L, et al. Long-term effects of an HIV/STI sexual risk reduction intervention for heterosexual couples. AIDS Behav 2005;9(1):1-13. PMID: 15812609. **KQ1E3, KQ2E3, KQ3E3, KQ4E3.**

68. El-Bassel N, Gilbert L, Wu E, et al. Couple-based HIV prevention for low-income drug users from New York City: a randomized controlled trial to reduce dual risks. J Acquir Immune Defic Syndr 2011 Oct 1;58(2):198-206. PMID: 21725249. **KQ1E2a, KQ2E2a, KQ3E2a, KQ4E2a.**

69. Enrhardt AA, Exner TM, Hoffman S, et al. HIV/STD risk and sexual strategies among women family planning clients in New York: Project FIO. AIDS Behav 2002;6(1):1-13. PMID: None. **KQ3E4, KQ4E4.**

70. Exner TM, Tesoriero JM, Battles HB, et al. A randomized controlled trial to evaluate a structural intervention to promote the female condom in New York state. AIDS & Behav 2012 Jul;16(5):1121-32. PMID: 22484992. **KQ1E1, KQ2E1, KQ3E1, KQ4E1.**

71. Ferrer RA, Fisher JD, Buck R, et al. Pilot test of an emotional education intervention component for sexual risk reduction. Health Psychol 2011 Sep;30(5):656-60. PMID: 21534680. **KQ1E2a, KQ2E2a, KQ3E2a, KQ4E2a.**

72. Flaskerud JH, Nyamathi AM, Uman GC. Longitudinal effects of an HIV testing and counseling programme for low-income Latina women. Ethn Health 1997 Mar;2(1-2):89-103. PMID: 10.1080/13557858.1997.9961818 [doi]. **KQ1E3, KQ2E3, KQ3E3, KQ4E3.**

73. Forehand R, Armistead L, Long N, et al. Efficacy of a parent-based sexual-risk prevention program for African American preadolescents: a randomized controlled trial. Arch Pediatr Adolesc Med 2007 Dec;161(12):1123-9. PMID: 18056556. **KQ1E2a, KQ2E2a, KQ3E2a, KQ4E2a.**

74. Fortune T, Wright E, Juzang I, et al. Recruitment, enrollment and retention of young black men for HIV prevention research: experiences from The 411 for Safe Text project. Contemp Clin Trials 2010 Mar;31(2):151-6. PMID: 20035899. **KQ1E2c, KQ2E2c, KQ3E2c, KQ4E2c.**

Appendix B. Excluded Studies

75. Gold J, Aitken CK, Dixon HG, et al. A randomised controlled trial using mobile advertising to promote safer sex and sun safety to young people. Health Educ Res 2011 Oct;26(5):782-94. PMID: 21447750. **KQ1E2c, KQ2E2c, KQ3E2c, KQ4E2c.**

76. Gollub EL, French P, Loundou A, et al. A randomized trial of hierarchical counseling in a short, clinic-based intervention to reduce the risk of sexually transmitted diseases in women. AIDS 2000 Jun 16;14(9):1249-55. **KQ1E3, KQ2E3, KQ3E3, KQ4E3.**

77. Gollub EL, Armstrong K, Boney T, et al. Correlates of trichomonas prevalence among street-recruited, drug-using women enrolled in a randomized trial. Subst Use Misuse 2010 Nov;45(13):2203-20. PMID: 20482337. **KQ1E2a, KQ2E2a, KQ3E2a, KQ4E2a.**

78. Gollub EL, Cyrus-Cameron E, Armstrong K, et al. Basic body knowledge in street-recruited, active drug-using women enrolled in a "body empowerment" intervention trial. AIDS Care 2012 Dec 7;25(6):732-7. PMID: 23216297. **KQ1E2a, KQ2E2a, KQ3E2a, KQ4E2a.**

79. Gottlieb SL, Douglas JM, Jr., Foster M, et al. Incidence of herpes simplex virus type 2 infection in 5 sexually transmitted disease (STD) clinics and the effect of HIV/STD risk-reduction counseling. J Infect Dis 2004 Sep 15;190(6):1059-67. PMID: 15319854. **KQ2E4, KQ3E4, KQ4E4.**

80. Grimley DM, Hook EW, III. A 15-minute interactive, computerized condom use intervention with biological endpoints. Sex Transm Dis 2009 Feb;36(2):73-8. PMID: 19125141. **KQ1E8a, KQ2E8a, KQ3E8a, KQ4E8a.**

81. Guilamo-Ramos V, Bouris A, Jaccard J, et al. A parent-based intervention to reduce sexual risk behavior in early adolescence: building alliances between physicians, social workers, and parents. J Adolesc Health 2011 Feb;48(2):159-63. PMID: 21257114. **KQ1E4, KQ3E4, KQ4E4.**

82. Harvey SM, Henderson JT, Thorburn S, et al. A randomized study of a pregnancy and disease prevention intervention for Hispanic couples. Perspect Sex Reprod Health 2004;36(4):162-9. PMID: 15321783. **KQ1E3, KQ2E3, KQ3E3, KQ4E3.**

83. Harvey SM, Kraft JM, West SG, et al. Effects of a health behavior change model--based HIV/STI prevention intervention on condom use among heterosexual couples: a randomized trial. Health Educ Behav 2009 Oct;36(5):878-94. PMID: 18784350. **KQ1E3, KQ2E3, KQ3E3, KQ4E3.**

84. Hien DA, Campbell AN, Killeen T, et al. The impact of trauma-focused group therapy upon HIV sexual risk behaviors in the NIDA Clinical Trials Network "Women and trauma" multi-site study. AIDS & Behav 2010 Apr;14(2):421-30. PMID: 19452271. **KQ1E2b, KQ2E2b, KQ3E2b, KQ4E2b.**

85. Hoffman JA, Klein H, Crosby H, et al. Project neighborhoods in action: an HIV-related intervention project targeting drug abusers in Washington, DC. J Urban Health 1999;76(4):419-34. PMID: 10609592. **KQ1E2a, KQ2E2a, KQ3E2a, KQ4E2a.**

86. Hoffman S, Exner TM, Leu CS, et al. Female-condom use in a gender-specific family planning clinic trial. Am J Public Health 2003 Nov;93(11):1897-903. PMID: 14600063. **KQ1E4, KQ3E4, KQ4E4.**

87. Holden AE, Shain RN, Miller WB, et al. The influence of depression on sexual risk reduction and STD infection in a controlled, randomized intervention trial. Sex Transm Dis 2008 Oct;35(10):898-904. PMID: 18607311. **KQ3E4, KQ4E4.**

88. Hops H, Ozechowski TJ, Waldron HB, et al. Adolescent health-risk sexual behaviors: effects of a drug abuse intervention. AIDS & Behav 2011 Nov;15(8):1664-76. PMID: 21833690. **KQ1E3, KQ2E3, KQ3E3, KQ4E3.**

89. Howard MN, Howard MN. Improving low-income teen health behaviors with Internet-linked clinic interventions. Sex Res Social Policy 2011 Mar;.8(1) PMID: None. **KQ1E8a, KQ2E8a, KQ3E8a, KQ4E8a.**

90. Imrie J, Stephenson JM, Cowan FM, et al. A cognitive behavioural intervention to reduce sexually transmitted infections among gay men: randomised trial. BMJ 2001 Jun 16;322(7300):1451-6. **KQ1E3, KQ2E3, KQ3E3, KQ4E3.**

91. Ito KE, Kalyanaraman S, Ford CA, et al. "Let's Talk About Sex": pilot study of an interactive CD-ROM to prevent HIV/STIS in female adolescents. AIDS Educ Prev 2008 Feb;20(1):78-89. PMID: 18312069. **KQ1E4, KQ2E4, KQ3E4, KQ4E4.**

Appendix B. Excluded Studies

92. Jemmott JB, III, Jemmott LS, Fong GT. Reductions in HIV risk-associated sexual behaviors among black male adolescents: effects of an AIDS prevention intervention. Am J Public Health 1992 Mar;82(3):372-7. PMID: 1536352. **KQ1E2a, KQ2E2a, KQ3E2a, KQ4E2a.**

93. Jemmott JB, III, Jemmott LS, Braverman PK, et al. HIV/STD risk reduction interventions for African American and Latino adolescent girls at an adolescent medicine clinic: a randomized controlled trial. Arch Pediatr Adolesc Med 2005 May;159(5):440-9. PMID: 15867118. **KQ3E4, KQ4E4.**

94. Jemmott JB, III, Jemmott LS, Fong GT, et al. Effectiveness of an HIV/STD risk-reduction intervention for adolescents when implemented by community-based organizations: a cluster-randomized controlled trial. Am J Public Health 2010 Apr;100(4):720-6. PMID: 20167903. **KQ1E2a, KQ2E2a, KQ3E2a, KQ4E2a.**

95. Jemmott LS, Jemmott JB, III, O'Leary A. Effects on sexual risk behavior and STD rate of brief HIV/STD prevention interventions for African American women in primary care settings. Am J Public Health 2007 Jun;97(6):1034-40. PMID: 17463391. **KQ3E4, KQ4E4.**

96. Jones DL, Kashy D, Villar-Loubet OM, et al. The impact of substance use, sexual trauma, and intimate partner violence on sexual risk intervention outcomes in couples: a randomized trial. Ann Behav Med 2012 Dec 4;45(3):318-28. PMID: 23208648. **KQ1E3, KQ2E3, KQ3E3, KQ4E3.**

97. Jones R, Lacroix LJ. Streaming weekly soap opera video episodes to smartphones in a randomized controlled trial to reduce HIV risk in young urban African American/black women. AIDS & Behav 2012 Jul;16(5):1341-58. PMID: 22430640. **KQ1E3, KQ2E3, KQ3E3, KQ4E3.**

98. Juzang I, Fortune T, Black S, et al. A pilot programme using mobile phones for HIV prevention. J Telemed Telecare 2011;17(3):150-3. PMID: 21270049. **KQ1E2c, KQ2E2c, KQ3E2c, KQ4E2c.**

99. Kalichman SC, Cain D, Weinhardt L, et al. Experimental components analysis of brief theory-based HIV/AIDS risk-reduction counseling for sexually transmitted infection patients. Health Psychol 2005 Mar;24(2):198-208. PMID: 15755234. **KQ1E3, KQ2E3, KQ3E3, KQ4E3.**

100. Kamb ML, Fishbein M, Douglas JM, Jr., et al. Efficacy of risk-reduction counseling to prevent human immunodeficiency virus and sexually transmitted diseases: a randomized controlled trial. Project RESPECT Study Group. JAMA 1998 Oct 7;280(13):1161-7. PMID: 9777816. **KQ3E4, KQ4E4.**

101. Kelly JA, McAuliffe TL, Sikkema KJ, et al. Reduction in risk behavior among adults with severe mental illness who learned to advocate for HIV prevention. J Consult Clin Psychol 1997;48(10):1283-8. PMID: 9323747. **KQ1E3, KQ2E3, KQ3E3, KQ4E3.**

102. Kennedy SB, Nolen S, Applewhite J, et al. Condom use behaviours among 18-24 year-old urban African American males: a qualitative study. AIDS Care 2007 Sep;19(8):1032-8. PMID: 17852001. **KQ1E2c, KQ2E2c, KQ3E2c, KQ4E2c.**

103. Kennedy SB, Nolen S, Applewhite J, et al. A quantitative study on the condom-use behaviors of eighteen- to twenty-four-year-old urban African American males. AIDS Patient Care STDS 2007 May;21(5):306-20. PMID: 17518523. **KQ1E2c, KQ2E2c, KQ3E2c, KQ4E2c.**

104. Kennedy SB, Nolen S, Pan Z, et al. Effectiveness of a brief condom promotion program in reducing risky sexual behaviours among African American men. J Eval Clin Pract 2012 Mar 21;19(2):408-13. PMID: 22435646. **KQ1E2c, KQ2E2c, KQ3E2c, KQ4E2c.**

105. Kershaw TS, Magriples U, Westdahl C, et al. Pregnancy as a window of opportunity for HIV prevention: effects of an HIV intervention delivered within prenatal care. Am J Public Health 2009 Nov;99(11):2079-86. PMID: 19762662. **KQ4E4.**

106. Klein CH, Card JJ. Preliminary efficacy of a computer-delivered HIV prevention intervention for African American teenage females. AIDS Educ Prev 2011 Dec;23(6):564-76. PMID: 22201239. **KQ1E2a, KQ2E2a, KQ3E2a, KQ4E2a.**

107. Koblin BA, Bonner S, Hoover DR, et al. A randomized trial of enhanced HIV risk-reduction and vaccine trial education interventions among HIV-negative, high-risk women who use noninjection drugs: the UNITY study. J Acquir Immune Defic Syndr 2010 Mar;53(3):378-87. PMID: 20190585. **KQ1E2a, KQ2E2a, KQ3E2a, KQ4E2a.**

Appendix B. Excluded Studies

108. Koblin BA, Bonner S, Powell B, et al. A randomized trial of a behavioral intervention for black MSM: the DiSH study. AIDS 2012 Feb 20;26(4):483-8. PMID: 22156967. **KQ1E5a, KQ2E5a, KQ3E5a, KQ4E5a.**

109. Kogan SM, Yu T, Brody GH, et al. Integrating condom skills into family-centered prevention: efficacy of the Strong African American Families-Teen program. J Adolesc Health 2012 Aug;51(2):164-70. PMID: 22824447. **KQ1E6, KQ2E6, KQ3E6, KQ4E6.**

110. Koniak-Griffin D, Lesser J, Takayanagi S, et al. Couple-focused human immunodeficiency virus prevention for young Latino parents: randomized clinical trial of efficacy and sustainability. Arch Pediatr Adolesc Med 2011 Apr;165(4):306-12. PMID: 21464378. **KQ1E3, KQ2E3, KQ3E3, KQ4E3.**

111. Konkle-Parker DJ, Amico KR, McKinney VE. Effects of an intervention addressing information, motivation, and behavioral skills on HIV care adherence in a southern clinic cohort. AIDS Care 2013 Oct 14 **KQ1E1, KQ2E1, KQ3E1, KQ4E1.**

112. Korte JE, Shain RN, Holden AE, et al. Reduction in sexual risk behaviors and infection rates among African Americans and Mexican Americans. Sex Transm Dis 2004 Mar;31(3):166-73. PMID: 15076930. **KQ3E4, KQ4E4.**

113. Kott A. Family intervention may reduce HIV risk-taking in Hispanic adolescents. [References]. Perspect Sex Reprod Health 2011 Dec;43(4):267-8. PMID: None. **KQ1E2c, KQ2E2c, KQ3E2c, KQ4E2c.**

114. Kraft JM, Harvey SM, Thorburn S, et al. Intervening with couples: assessing contraceptive outcomes in a randomized pregnancy and HIV/STD risk reduction intervention trial. Womens Health Issues 2007 Jan;17(1):52-60. PMID: 17321948. **KQ1E3, KQ2E3, KQ3E3, KQ4E3.**

115. Kurtz SP, Stall RD, Buttram ME, et al. A randomized trial of a behavioral intervention for high risk substance-using MSM. AIDS Behav 2013 Jun 4 PMID: 23732957. **KQ1E5a, KQ2E5a, KQ3E5a, KQ4E5a.**

116. Lang DL, DiClemente RJ, Hardin JW, et al. Threats of cross-contamination on effects of a sexual risk reduction intervention: fact or fiction. Prev Sci 2009 Sep;10(3):270-5. PMID: 19241171. **KQ1E4, KQ4E4.**

117. Lau JT, Lau M, Cheung A, et al. A randomized controlled study to evaluate the efficacy of an Internet-based intervention in reducing HIV risk behaviors among men who have sex with men in Hong Kong. AIDS Care 2008 Aug;20(7):820-8. PMID: 18608057. **KQ1E2c, KQ2E2c, KQ3E2c, KQ4E2c.**

118. Lau JT, Tsui HY, Cheng S, et al. A randomized controlled trial to evaluate the relative efficacy of adding voluntary counseling and testing (VCT) to information dissemination in reducing HIV-related risk behaviors among Hong Kong male cross-border truck drivers. AIDS Care 2010 Jan;22(1):17-28. PMID: 20390477. **KQ1E2a, KQ2E2a, KQ3E2a, KQ4E2a.**

119. Lau JT, Tsui HY. Voluntary counselling and testing plus information distribution to reduce HIV-related risk behaviours among Hong Kong male cross-border truck drivers: a randomised controlled study. Hong Kong Med J 2012 Aug;18(Suppl 3):39-41. PMID: 22865223. **KQ1E2a, KQ2E2a, KQ3E2a, KQ4E2a.**

120. Lau JT, Tsui HY, Lau MM. A pilot clustered randomized control trial evaluating the efficacy of a network-based HIV peer-education intervention targeting men who have sex with men in Hong Kong, China. AIDS Care 2012 Dec 17;25(7):812-9. PMID: 23244706. **KQ1E6, KQ2E6, KQ3E6, KQ4E6.**

121. Lesser J, Koniak-Griffin D, Huang R, et al. Parental protectiveness and unprotected sexual activity among Latino adolescent mothers and fathers. AIDS Educ Prev 2009 Oct;21(5:Suppl):88-102. PMID: 19824837. **KQ1E3, KQ2E3, KQ3E3, KQ4E3.**

122. Li X, Stanton B, Feigelman S, et al. Unprotected sex among African-American adolescents a three-year study. J Natl Med Assoc 2002;94(9):789-96. PMID: 12392042. **KQ1E2a, KQ2E2a, KQ3E2a, KQ4E2a.**

123. Lindenberg CS, Solorzano RM, Bear D, et al. Reducing substance use and risky sexual behavior among young, low-income, Mexican-American women: comparison of two interventions. Appl Nurs Res 2002;15(3):137-48. PMID: 12173165. **KQ1E8b, KQ2E8b, KQ3E8b, KQ4E8b.**

Appendix B. Excluded Studies

124. Mallory C, Hesson-McInnis M. Pilot test results of an HIV prevention intervention for high-risk women. West J Nurs Res 2013 Mar;35(3):313-29. PMID: 21827425. **KQ1E8a, KQ2E8a, KQ3E8a, KQ4E8a.**

125. Malow RM, McMahon RC, Devieux J, et al. Cognitive behavioral HIV risk reduction in those receiving psychiatric treatment: a clinical trial. AIDS & Behav 2012 Jul;16(5):1192-202. PMID: 22210481. **KQ1E5b, KQ2E5b, KQ3E5b, KQ4E5b.**

126. Mansergh G, Koblin BA, McKirnan DJ, et al. An intervention to reduce HIV risk behavior of substance-using men who have sex with men: a two-group randomized trial with a nonrandomized third group. PLoS Med 2010;7(8):e1000329. PMID: 20811491. **KQ1E5b, KQ2E5b, KQ3E5b, KQ4E5b.**

127. Marion LN, Finnegan L, Campbell RT, et al. The Well Woman Program: a community-based randomized trial to prevent sexually transmitted infections in low-income African American women. Res Nurs Health 2009 Jun;32(3):274-85. PMID: 19373824. **KQ3E4.**

128. Marrazzo JM, Thomas KK, Fiedler TL, et al. Relationship of specific vaginal bacteria and bacterial vaginosis treatment failure in women who have sex with women. Ann Intern Med 2008 Jul 1;149(1):20-8. PMID: 18591634. **KQ2E4, KQ3E4, KQ4E4.**

129. Marrazzo JM, Thomas KK, Agnew K, et al. Prevalence and risks for bacterial vaginosis in women who have sex with women. Sex Transm Dis 2010 May;37(5):335-9. PMID: 20429087. **KQ2E4, KQ3E4, KQ4E4.**

130. Marrazzo JM, Thomas KK, Ringwood K. A behavioural intervention to reduce persistence of bacterial vaginosis among women who report sex with women: results of a randomised trial. Sex Transm Infect 2011 Aug;87(5):399-405. PMID: 21653935. **KQ2E4, KQ3E4, KQ4E4.**

131. Marsch LA, Grabinski MJ, Bickel WK, et al. Computer-assisted HIV prevention for youth with substance use disorders. Subst Use Misuse 2011;46(1):46-56. PMID: 21190405. **KQ1E2b, KQ2E2b, KQ3E2b, KQ4E2b.**

132. Mausbach BT, Semple SJ, Strathdee SA, et al. Efficacy of a behavioral intervention for increasing safer sex behaviors in HIV-negative, heterosexual methamphetamine users: results from the Fast-Lane Study. Ann Behav Med 2007 Nov;34(3):263-74. PMID: 18020936. **KQ1E2c, KQ2E2c, KQ3E2c, KQ4E2c.**

133. McCollister KE, Freitas DM, Prado G, et al. Opportunity Costs and Financial Incentives for Hispanic Youth Participating in a Family-Based HIV and Substance Use Preventive Intervention. J Prim Prev 2013 Oct 26 **KQ1E2a, KQ2E2a, KQ3E2a, KQ4E2a.**

134. McCoy CB, Chitwood DD, Khoury EL. The implementation of an experimental research design in the evaluation of an intervention to prevent AIDS among IV drug users. J Drug Issues 1990;20(2):215-22. PMID: None. **KQ1E4, KQ2E4, KQ3E4, KQ4E4.**

135. McCoy HV, Dodds SE, Nolan C. AIDS intervention design for program evaluation: the Miami Community Outreach Program. J Drug Issues 1990;20(2):223-43. PMID: None. **KQ1E4, KQ2E4, KQ3E4, KQ4E4.**

136. McMahon JM, Tortu S, Pouget ER, et al. Effectiveness of couple-based HIV counseling and testing for women substance users and their primary male partners: a randomized trial. Adv Prev Med 2013;2013:286207. PMID: 23555059. **KQ1E2c, KQ2E2c, KQ3E2c, KQ4E2c.**

137. Melendez RM, Hoffman S, Exner T, et al. Intimate partner violence and safer sex negotiation: effects of a gender-specific intervention. Arch Sex Behav 2003 Dec;32(6):499-511. PMID: 14574094. **KQ1E4, KQ4E4.**

138. Metsch LR, Feaster DJ, Gooden L, et al. Implementing rapid HIV testing with or without risk-reduction counseling in drug treatment centers: results of a randomized trial. Am J Public Health 2012 Jun;102(6):1160-7. PMID: 22515871. **KQ1E2b, KQ2E2b, KQ3E2b, KQ4E2b.**

139. Metsch LR, Feaster DJ, Gooden L, et al. Effect of risk-reduction counseling with rapid HIV testing on risk of acquiring sexually transmitted infections: the AWARE randomized controlled trial. JAMA 2013;310(16):1701-10. PMID: 24150466. **KQ3E4.**

Appendix B. Excluded Studies

140. Mevissen FE, Ruiter RA, Meertens RM, et al. Justify your love: testing an online STI-risk communication intervention designed to promote condom use and STI-testing. Psychol Health 2011 Feb;26(2):205-21. PMID: 21318930. **KQ1E2c, KQ2E2c, KQ3E2c, KQ4E2c.**

141. Milhausen RR, DiClemente RJ, Lang DL, et al. Frequency of sex after an intervention to decrease sexual risk-taking among African-American adolescent girls: Results of a randomized, controlled clinical trial. Sex Education 2008;8:47-57. **KQ1E4, KQ3E4, KQ4E4.**

142. Milhausen RR, Milhausen RR. Justify your love: testing an online STI-risk communication intervention designed to promote condom use and STI-testing. Sex Educ 2008 Feb;8(1):47-57. PMID: None. **KQ1E4, KQ3E4, KQ4E4.**

143. Miller KS, Forehand R, Wiegand R, et al. Making HIV prevention programming count: identifying predictors of success in a parent-based HIV prevention program for youth. AIDS Educ Prev 2011 Feb;23(1):38-53. PMID: 21341959. **KQ1E4, KQ2E4, KQ3E4, KQ4E4.**

144. Miller KS, Lin CY, Poulsen MN, et al. Enhancing HIV communication between parents and children: efficacy of the Parents Matter! Program. AIDS Educ Prev 2011 Dec;23(6):550-63. PMID: 22201238. **KQ1E4, KQ2E4, KQ3E4, KQ4E4.**

145. Miller S, Exner TM, Williams SP, et al. A gender-specific intervention for at-risk women in the USA. AIDS Care 2000 Oct;12(5):603-12. PMID: 11218546. **KQ1E4, KQ3E4, KQ4E4.**

146. Mimiaga MJ, Noonan E, Donnell D, et al. Childhood sexual abuse is highly associated with HIV risk-taking behavior and infection among MSM in the EXPLORE Study. J Acquir Immune Defic Syndr 2009 Jul 1;51(3):340-8. PMID: 19367173. **KQ1E2a, KQ2E2a, KQ3E2a, KQ4E2a.**

147. Mittal M, Senn TE, Carey MP. Mediators of the relation between partner violence and sexual risk behavior among women attending a sexually transmitted disease clinic. Sex Transm Dis 2011 Jun;38(6):510-5. PMID: 21258269. **KQ3E4.**

148. Morgenstern J, Bux DA, Jr., Parsons J, et al. Randomized trial to reduce club drug use and HIV risk behaviors among men who have sex with men. J Consult Clin Psychol 2009 Aug;77(4):645-56. PMID: 19634958. **KQ1E5a, KQ2E5a, KQ3E5a, KQ4E5a.**

149. Morrison-Beedy D, Carey MP, Kowalski J, et al. Group-based HIV risk reduction intervention for adolescent girls: evidence of feasibility and efficacy. Res Nurs Health 2005 Feb;28(1):3-15. PMID: 15625713. **KQ1E8a, KQ2E8a, KQ3E8a, KQ4E8a.**

150. Morrison-Beedy D, Carey MP, Crean HF, et al. Determinants of adolescent female attendance at an HIV risk reduction program. J Assoc Nurses AIDS Care 2010 Mar;21(2):153-61. PMID: 20116296. **KQ1E2a, KQ2E2a, KQ3E2a, KQ4E2a.**

151. Morrison-Beedy D, Jones SH, Xia Y, et al. Reducing sexual risk behavior in adolescent girls: results from a randomized controlled trial. J Adolesc Health 2013 Mar;52(3):314-21. PMID: 23299011. **KQ1E2a, KQ2E2a, KQ3E2a, KQ4E2a.**

152. Murry VM, Berkel C, Chen YF, et al. Intervention induced changes on parenting practices, youth self-pride and sexual norms to reduce HIV-related behaviors among rural African American youths. J Youth Adolesc 2011 Sep;40(9):1147-63. PMID: 21373904. **KQ1E2a, KQ2E2a, KQ3E2a, KQ4E2a.**

153. Mustanski B, Garofalo R, Monahan C, et al. Feasibility, acceptability, and preliminary efficacy of an online HIV prevention program for diverse young men who have sex with men: the Keep It Up! intervention. AIDS Behav 2013 May 15 PMID: 23673793. **KQ1E3, KQ2E3, KQ3E3, KQ4E3.**

154. Negash S. Sexual health education in college: The impact of sexual negotiation training on sexual risk reduction. Dissertation Abstracts International Section A: Humanities and Social Sciences. 2013;74:No. **KQ1E2c, KQ2E2c, KQ3E2c, KQ4E2c.**

155. Neumann MS, O'Donnell L, Doval AS, et al. Effectiveness of the VOICES/VOCES sexually transmitted disease/human immunodeficiency virus prevention intervention when administered by health department staff: does it work in the "real world"? Sex Transm Dis 2011 Feb;38(2):133-9. PMID: 20729794. **KQ2E4, KQ3E4, KQ4E4.**

Appendix B. Excluded Studies

156. NIMH Collaborative HIV/STD Prevention Trial Group. Results of the NIMH collaborative HIV/sexually transmitted disease prevention trial of a community popular opinion leader intervention. J Acquir Immune Defic Syndr 2010 Jun;54(2):204-14. PMID: 20354444. **KQ1E10, KQ2E10, KQ3E10, KQ4E10.**

157. Norr KF, Ferrer L, Cianelli R, et al. Peer group intervention for HIV prevention among health workers in Chile. J Assoc Nurses AIDS Care 2012 Jan;23(1):73-86. PMID: 21497113. **KQ1E2a, KQ2E2a, KQ3E2a, KQ4E2a.**

158. Norton W, Fisher J, Amico K, et al. Relative efficacy of a pregnancy, sexually transmitted infection, or human immunodeficiency virus prevention-focused intervention on changing sexual risk behavior among young adults. J Am Coll Health 2012 Nov;60(8):574-82. PMID: 23157199. **KQ1E2c, KQ2E2c, KQ3E2c, KQ4E2c.**

159. Nydegger LA, Keeler AR, Hood C, et al. Effects of a one-hour intervention on condom implementation intentions among drug users in Southern California. AIDS Care 2013 May 8 PMID: 23656365. **KQ1E2c, KQ2E2c, KQ3E2c, KQ4E2c.**

160. O'Leary A, Jemmott LS, Jemmott JB. Mediation analysis of an effective sexual risk-reduction intervention for women: the importance of self-efficacy. Health Psychol 2008 Mar;27(2 Suppl):S180-S184. PMID: 18377160. **KQ3E4, KQ4E4.**

161. Pachankis JE, Lelutiu-Weinberger C, Golub SA, et al. Developing an online health intervention for young gay and bisexual Men. AIDS Behav 2013 May 15 PMID: 23673791. **KQ1E4, KQ2E4, KQ3E4, KQ4E4.**

162. Pantin H, Prado G, Lopez B, et al. A randomized controlled trial of Familias Unidas for Hispanic adolescents with behavior problems. Psychosom Med 2009 Nov;71(9):987-95. PMID: 19834053. **KQ1E2a, KQ2E2a, KQ3E2a, KQ4E2a.**

163. Peipert J, Redding CA, Blume J, et al. Design of a stage-matched intervention trial to increase dual method contraceptive use (Project PROTECT). Contemp Clin Trials 2007 Sep;28(5):626-37. PMID: 17374567. **KQ4E4.**

164. Peipert JF, Redding CA, Blume JD, et al. Tailored intervention to increase dual-contraceptive method use: a randomized trial to reduce unintended pregnancies and sexually transmitted infections. Am J Obstet Gynecol 2008 Jun;198(6):630-8. PMID: 18395692. **KQ4E4.**

165. Peragallo N, Gonzalez-Guarda RM, McCabe BE, et al. The efficacy of an HIV risk reduction intervention for Hispanic women. AIDS & Behav 2012 Jul;16(5):1316-26. PMID: 21969175. **KQ1E2a, KQ2E2a, KQ3E2a, KQ4E2a.**

166. Pereira LM. Risk and relationship: examining the outcomes of couples-based HIV prevention among low-income men of color in heterosexual relationships. New York: Columbia University; 2001. PMID: None. **KQ1E3, KQ2E3, KQ3E3, KQ4E3.**

167. Peterman A. Physician initiated STI prevention counselling: targeting women to reach couples. Ontario: University of Western Ontario; 2008. PMID: None. **KQ1E12, KQ2E12, KQ3E12, KQ4E12.**

168. Petersen R, Albright J, Garrett JM, et al. Pregnancy and STD prevention counseling using an adaptation of motivational interviewing: a randomized controlled trial. Perspect Sex Reprod Health 2007 Mar;39(1):21-8. PMID: 17335378. **KQ2E4, KQ4E4.**

169. Picciano JF, Roffman RA, Kalichman SC, et al. Lowering obstacles to HIV prevention services: effects of a brief, telephone-based intervention using motivational enhancement therapy. Ann Behav Med 2007 Oct;34(2):177-87. PMID: 17927556. **KQ1E2c, KQ2E2c, KQ3E2c, KQ4E2c.**

170. Prado G, Pantin H, Briones E, et al. A randomized controlled trial of a parent-centered intervention in preventing substance use and HIV risk behaviors in Hispanic adolescents. J Consult Clin Psychol 2007 Dec;75(6):914-26. PMID: 18085908. **KQ1E2a, KQ2E2a, KQ3E2a, KQ4E2a.**

171. Prado G, Pantin H, Huang S, et al. Effects of a family intervention in reducing HIV risk behaviors among high-risk Hispanic adolescents: a randomized controlled trial. Arch Pediatr Adolesc Med 2012 Feb;166(2):127-33. PMID: 21969363. **KQ1E2c, KQ2E2c, KQ3E2c, KQ4E2c.**

Appendix B. Excluded Studies

172. Proude EM, D'Este C, Ward JE. Randomized trial in family practice of a brief intervention to reduce STI risk in young adults. Fam Pract 2004 Oct;21(5):537-44. PMID: 15367476. **KQ1E4, KQ3E4, KQ4E4.**

173. Reback CJ, Peck JA, Dierst-Davies R, et al. Contingency management among homeless, out-of-treatment men who have sex with men. J Subst Abuse Treat 2010 Oct;39(3):255-63. PMID: 20667681. **KQ1E5a, KQ2E5a, KQ3E5a, KQ4E5a.**

174. Rhodes F, Stein JA, Fishbein M, et al. Using theory to understand how interventions work: Project RESPECT, condom use, and the Integrative Model. AIDS & Behav 2007 May;11(3):393-407. PMID: 17323123. **KQ3E4, KQ4E4.**

175. Rhodes SD, McCoy TP, Vissman AT, et al. A randomized controlled trial of a culturally congruent intervention to increase condom use and HIV testing among heterosexually active immigrant Latino men. AIDS & Behav 2011 Nov;15(8):1764-75. PMID: 21301948. **KQ1E2a, KQ2E2a, KQ3E2a, KQ4E2a.**

176. Rosser BR, Oakes JM, Konstan J, et al. Reducing HIV risk behavior of men who have sex with men through persuasive computing: results of the Men's INTernet Study-II. AIDS 2010 Aug 24;24(13):2099-107. PMID: 20601853. **KQ1E2c, KQ2E2c, KQ3E2c, KQ4E2c.**

177. Rosser BRS. Evaluation of the efficacy of AIDS education interventions for homosexually active men. Health Educ Res 1990;5(3):299-308. PMID: None. **KQ1E2c, KQ2E2c, KQ3E2c, KQ4E2c.**

178. Rotheram-Borus MJ. HIV prevention in persons with mental health problems. Psychol Health Med 2006;11(2):142-54. PMID: 17129904. **KQ1E3, KQ2E3, KQ3E3, KQ4E3.**

179. Roye C, Perlmutter SP, Krauss B. A brief, low-cost, theory-based intervention to promote dual method use by black and Latina female adolescents: a randomized clinical trial. Health Educ Behav 2007 Aug;34(4):608-21. PMID: 16740522. **KQ1E8a, KQ2E8a, KQ3E8a, KQ4E8a.**

180. Sales JM, Lang DL, Hardin JW, et al. Efficacy of an HIV prevention program among African American female adolescents reporting high depressive symptomatology. J Womens Health (Larchmt) 2010 Feb;19(2):219-27. PMID: 20109119. **KQ1E4, KQ3E4, KQ4E4.**

181. Sales JM, Lang DL, DiClemente RJ, et al. The mediating role of partner communication frequency on condom use among African American adolescent females participating in an HIV prevention intervention. Health Psychol 2012 Jan;31(1):63-9. PMID: 21843001. **KQ1E3, KQ2E3, KQ3E3, KQ4E3.**

182. Sanchez J, De La Rosa M, Serna CA. Project Salud: Efficacy of a Community-Based HIV Prevention Intervention for Hispanic Migrant Workers in South Florida. AIDS Education & Prevention 2013 Oct;25(5):363-75. **KQ1E2c, KQ2E2c, KQ3E2c, KQ4E2c.**

183. Sanderson CA, Yopyk DJ. Improving condom use intentions and behavior by changing perceived partner norms: an evaluation of condom promotion videos for college students. Health Psychol 2007 Jul;26(4):481-7. PMID: 17605568. **KQ1E2a, KQ2E2a, KQ3E2a, KQ4E2a.**

184. Scholes D, McBride CM, Grothaus L, et al. A tailored minimal self-help intervention to promote condom use in young women: results from a randomized trial. AIDS 2003 Jul 4;17(10):1547-56. PMID: 12824793. **KQ3E4, KQ4E4.**

185. Schumann A, Nyamathi A, Stein JA. HIV risk reduction in a nurse case-managed TB and HIV intervention among homeless adults. J Health Psychol 2007 Sep;12(5):833-43. PMID: 17855466. **KQ1E2a, KQ2E2a, KQ3E2a, KQ4E2a.**

186. Schwartz RP, Stitzer ML, Feaster DJ, et al. HIV rapid testing in drug treatment: comparison across treatment modalities. J Subst Abuse Treat 2013 Apr;44(4):369-74. PMID: 23021496. **KQ1E2b, KQ2E2b, KQ3E2b, KQ4E2b.**

187. Seibold-Simpson S, Morrison-Beedy D. Avoiding early study attrition in adolescent girls: impact of recruitment contextual factors. West J Nurs Res 2010 Oct;32(6):761-78. PMID: 20634400. **KQ1E2a, KQ2E2a, KQ3E2a, KQ4E2a.**

Appendix B. Excluded Studies

188. Semaan S, Neumann MS, Hutchins K, et al. Brief counseling for reducing sexual risk and bacterial STIs among drug users--results from project RESPECT. Drug Alcohol Depend 2010 Jan 1;106(1):7-15. PMID: 19720471., **KQ3E4, KQ4E4.**

189. Senn N, de VS, Berdoz D, et al. Motivational brief intervention for the prevention of sexually transmitted infections in travelers: a randomized controlled trial. BMC Infect Dis 2011;11:300. PMID: 22044609. **KQ1E8c, KQ2E8c, KQ3E8c, KQ4E8c.**

190. Shain RN, Piper JM, Newton ER, et al. Even if you build it, we may not come: correlates of non-attendance at a sexual risk reduction workshop for STD clinic patients. N Engl J Med 1999 Jan 14;340(2):93-100. PMID: 9887160**KQ3E4, KQ4E4.**

191. Shain RN, Piper JM, Holden AE, et al. Prevention of gonorrhea and Chlamydia through behavioral intervention: results of a two-year controlled randomized trial in minority women. Sex Transm Dis 2004 Jul;31(7):401-8. PMID: 15215694. **KQ3E4, KQ4E4.**

192. Shoptaw S, Reback CJ, Larkins S, et al. Outcomes using two tailored behavioral treatments for substance abuse in urban gay and bisexual men. J Subst Abuse Treat 2008 Oct;35(3):285-93. PMID: 18329226. **KQ1E3, KQ2E3, KQ3E3, KQ4E3.**

193. Sieving RE, Bernat DH, Resnick MD, et al. A clinic-based youth development program to reduce sexual risk behaviors among adolescent girls: prime time pilot study. Health Promot Pract 2012 Jul;13(4):462-71. PMID: 21606323. **KQ1E1, KQ2E1, KQ3E1, KQ4E1.**

194. Sinclair AH, Tolsma D, Weathersby A, et al. Feasibility of conducting a large, randomized controlled trial for STD counseling in a managed care setting. Sex Transm Dis 2008 Nov;35(11):920-3. PMID: 18665018. **KQ1E4, KQ2E4, KQ3E4, KQ4E4.**

195. Slesnick N, Kang MJ. The impact of an integrated treatment on HIV risk behavior among homeless youth: a randomized controlled trial. J Behav Med 2008 Feb;31(1):45-59. PMID: 17940861. **KQ1E2a, KQ2E2a, KQ3E2a, KQ4E2a.**

196. Smith PB, Weinman ML, Parrilli J. The role of condom motivation education in the reduction of new and reinfection rates of sexually transmitted diseases among inner-city female adolescents. Patient Educ Couns 1997 May;31(1):77-81. PMID: S0738-3991(97)01009-4 [pii]. **KQ1E8b, KQ2E8b, KQ3E8b, KQ4E8b.**

197. St Lawrence JS, Brasfield TL, Jefferson KW, et al. Cognitive-behavioral intervention to reduce African American adolescents' risk for HIV infection. J Consult Clin Psychol 1995;63(2):221-37. PMID: 7751483. **KQ1E3, KQ2E3, KQ3E3, KQ4E3.**

198. Sullivan PS, White D, Rosenberg ES, et al. Safety and acceptability of couples HIV testing and counseling for US men who have sex with men: a randomized prevention study. J Int Assoc Provid AIDS Care 2013 Aug 30 PMID: 23995295. **KQ1E3, KQ2E3, KQ3E3, KQ4E3.**

199. Swartz LH, Sherman CA, Harvey SM, et al. Midlife women online: evaluation of an internet-based program to prevent unintended pregnancy & STIs. J Women Aging 2011;23(4):342-59. PMID: 22014222. **KQ1E2c, KQ2E2c, KQ3E2c, KQ4E2c.**

200. Thurman AR, Holden AE, Shain RN, et al. Preventing recurrent sexually transmitted diseases in minority adolescents: a randomized controlled trial. Obstet Gynecol 2008 Jun;111(6):1417-25. PMID: 18515527. **KQ3E4, KQ4E4.**

201. Thurman AR, Holden AE, Shain RN, et al. The male sexual partners of adult versus teen women with sexually transmitted infections. Sex Transm Dis 2009 Dec;36(12):768-74. PMID: 19704393. **KQ1E7, KQ2E7, KQ3E7, KQ4E7.**

202. Tobin K, Kuramoto SJ, German D, et al. Unity in Diversity: results of a randomized clinical culturally tailored pilot HIV prevention intervention trial in Baltimore, Maryland, for African American men who have sex with men. Health Educ Behav 2012 Sep 14 PMID: 22984216. **KQ1E5a, KQ2E5a, KQ3E5a, KQ4E5a.**

203. Tobin KE, Kuramoto SJ, Davey-Rothwell MA, et al. The STEP into Action study: a peer-based, personal risk network-focused HIV prevention intervention with injection drug users in Baltimore, Maryland. Addiction 2011 Feb;106(2):366-75. PMID: 21054614. **KQ1E6, KQ2E6, KQ3E6, KQ4E6.**

Appendix B. Excluded Studies

204. Tolou-Shams M, Houck C, Conrad SM, et al. HIV prevention for juvenile drug court offenders: a randomized controlled trial focusing on affect management. J Correct Health Care 2011 Jul;17(3):226-32. PMID: 21474529. **KQ1E2a, KQ2E2a, KQ3E2a, KQ4E2a.**

205. Trenholm C, Devaney B, Fortson K, et al. Impacts of abstinence education on teen sexual activity, risk of pregnancy, and risk of sexually transmitted diseases. J Policy Anal Manage 2008;27(2):255-76. PMID: 18401923. **KQ1E2a, KQ2E2a, KQ3E2a, KQ4E2a.**

206. Tross S, Campbell AN, Cohen LR, et al. Effectiveness of HIV/STD sexual risk reduction groups for women in substance abuse treatment programs: results of NIDA Clinical Trials Network Trial. J Acquir Immune Defic Syndr 2008 Aug 15;48(5):581-9. PMID: 18645513. **KQ1E2b, KQ2E2b, KQ3E2b, KQ4E2b.**

207. Warner L, Klausner JD, Rietmeijer CA, et al. Effect of a brief video intervention on incident infection among patients attending sexually transmitted disease clinics. PLoS Med 2008 Jun 24;5(6):e135. PMID: 18578564. **KQ2E4, KQ3E4, KQ4E4.**

208. Weir BW, O'Brien K, Bard RS, et al. Reducing HIV and partner violence risk among women with criminal justice system involvement: a randomized controlled trial of two motivational interviewing-based interventions. AIDS Behav 2009 Jun;13(3):509-22. PMID: 18636325. **KQ1E5b, KQ2E5b, KQ3E5b, KQ4E5b.**

209. Wenger NS, Greenberg JM, Hilborne LH, et al. Effect of HIV antibody testing and AIDS education on communication about HIV risk and sexual behavior. A randomized, controlled trial in college students. Ann Intern Med 1992 Dec 1;117(11):905-11. PMID: 1443951. **KQ1E4, KQ3E4, KQ4E4.**

210. Wilson TE, Hogben M, Malka ES, et al. A randomized controlled trial for reducing risks for sexually transmitted infections through enhanced patient-based partner notification. Am J Public Health 2009 Apr;99:Suppl-10. PMID: 18556619. **KQ1E6, KQ2E6, KQ3E6, KQ4E6.**

211. Wilton L, Herbst JH, Coury-Doniger P, et al. Efficacy of an HIV/STI prevention intervention for black men who have sex with men: findings from the Many Men, Many Voices (3MV) project. AIDS & Behav 2009 Jun;13(3):532-44. PMID: 19267264. **KQ1E6, KQ2E6, KQ3E6, KQ4E6.**

212. Wingood GM, DiClemente RJ, Harrington KF, et al. Efficacy of an HIV prevention program among female adolescents experiencing gender-based violence. Am J Public Health 2006 Jun;96(6):1085-90. PMID: 16670238. **KQ4E4.**

213. Wingood GM, Card JJ, Er D, et al. Preliminary efficacy of a computer-based HIV intervention for African-American women. Psychol Health 2011 Feb;26(2):223-34. PMID: 21318931. **KQ1E3, KQ2E3, KQ3E3, KQ4E3.**

214. Wingood GM, DiClemente RJ, Villamizar K, et al. Efficacy of a health educator-delivered HIV prevention intervention for Latina women: a randomized controlled trial. Am J Public Health 2011 Dec;101(12):2245-52. PMID: 22021297. **KQ1E3, KQ2E3, KQ3E3, KQ4E3.**

215. Wingood GM, DiClemente RJ, Robinson-Simpson L, et al. Efficacy of an HIV intervention in reducing high-risk human papillomavirus, nonviral sexually transmitted infections, and concurrency among African American women: a randomized-controlled trial. JAIDS 2013 Jun 1;63(Suppl 1):S36-S43. PMID: 23673884. **KQ2E8b, KQ3E4, KQ4E4.**

216. Witte SS, El-Bassel N, Gilbert L, et al. Promoting female condom use to heterosexual couples: findings from a randomized clinical trial. Perspect Sex Reprod Health 2006;38(3):148-54. PMID: 16963388. **KQ1E3, KQ2E3, KQ3E3, KQ4E3.**

217. Yancey EM, Mayberry R, Armstrong-Mensah E, et al. The community-based participatory intervention effect of "HIV-RAAP". Am J Health Behav 2012 Jul;36(4):555-68. PMID: 22488405. **KQ1E2a, KQ2E2a, KQ3E2a, KQ4E2a.**

218. Zule WA, Bobashev GV, Reif SM, et al. Results of a pilot test of a brief computer-assisted tailored HIV prevention intervention for use with a range of demographic and risk groups. AIDS Behav 2013 Jul 20 PMID: 23872994. **KQ1E2b, KQ2E2b, KQ3E2b, KQ4E2b.**

Appendix C Table 1. Intervention Characteristics of Included Studies Targeting Adolescents

Author, year	Intervention	Description	Delivery and Format Method	No. of Sessions	Duration of Intervention	Provider
Boekeloo, 1999[63,143]	ASSESS (Awareness, Skills, Self-efficacy/Self-esteem, and Social Support)	An educational program targeting physicians and adolescents provided comprehensive HIV/STI prevention information, based on social cognitive theory and theory of reasoned action. Program aimed to increase adolescent awareness about sexual risks, skills to avoid risky sexual situations, self-efficacy (e.g., feeling that peer pressure can be resisted), and social support (such that adolescents felt encouraged by the physician). 15-min audiotaped risk assessment and education program (addressed awareness and perceived susceptibility to STIs); physician review of risk assessment and discussion, with props and brochures covering skills and self-efficacy to resist intercourse or use condoms, community resources, and (for parents) how to discuss sexual risks with teens.	Individual, face-to-face, video and print	1	Once	Primary care physicians, including a pediatrician
	Usual care	General health examination with no risk assessment and educational tools provided at time of visit.	Individual, face-to-face	1	Once	Pediatrician
Champion, 2012[69]	AIDS risk reduction	All participants received enhanced clinical counseling that included asking participants if they took all their medicine, had sex before completing treatment, their partner was treated, and if they had sex with him either before or during treatment. Physical exam and semi-structured one-to-one interview at entry, 6- and 12-month followup (1.5 to 2 hr), two workshop sessions initiated 1 to 3 weeks after entry (4 to 8 participants, 3 to 4 hr, one per week), conducted in round table format using motivational interviewing principles. Session 1 (awareness and perception of risk): raise awareness of personal risk, illustrate risks, discuss general STI and transmission routes, discuss selection of sex partners, discuss unintended pregnancy. Session 2 (commitment to change, strategies to reduce risk behavior): discuss how STIs and unintended pregnancy can be prevented, discussion with sex partner, importance of completing STI treatment, reflect on romantic relationships, share sexual decisionmaking skills, empathize how behavior can change participant life, discuss how to find support, reflect on knowledge and goals. Problem solving followup visits as needed. Weekly (3 to 5) support group sessions started 1 week after completion of both workshops. Two or more individual counseling sessions as initiated by participant to focus on expressed needs.	Individual and group, face-to-face	11	3 weeks (workshops only)	Nurse practitioner
	Minimal intervention	Enhanced clinical counseling included asking participants if they took all their medicine, had sex before completing treatment, their partner was treated, and if they had sex with him either before or during treatment. Participants told they can receive counseling intervention at study completion. Workshop and support group sessions provided to CG identical to those for IG and conducted by same facilitator, without an incentive.	Individual, face-to-face	1	Once	Nurse practitioner

Appendix C Table 1. Intervention Characteristics of Included Studies Targeting Adolescents

Author, year	Intervention	Description	Delivery and Format Method	No. of Sessions	Duration of Intervention	Provider
Danielson, 1990[66]	Reproductive health consultation	Slide tape program (30 min) with photos and information on sexual health, couple communication, and access to health services; visit with health practitioner (30 min), Q&A based on patient's interests, risk reduction counseling, modeling and rehearsing discussing sex and contraception with girlfriend	Individual, face-to-face	1	Once	Trained nurse practitioner, physician assistant or registered nurse
	Waitlist	Scheduled consultation after 12 months	NA	NA	NA	NA
DiClemente, 2004[68,148-153]	HIV prevention	Four 4-hr interactive group sessions implemented on consecutive Saturdays at a family clinic; 10 to 12 participants per group. Implemented by a trained African American female health educator and two African American female peer educators. Content based on social cognitive theory and theory of gender and power. Session 1: ethnic and gender pride; session 2: enhanced awareness of HIV risk reduction strategies (abstinence, consistent condom use, fewer sex partners); session 3: role play and cognitive rehearsal to enhance confidence in initiating safer-sex conversations, negotiating safer sex, refusing unsafe sex, and modeling condom use; session 4: importance of healthy relationships	Group, face-to-face	4	4 weeks	Trained health and peer educators
	Attention control	Four 4-hr interactive group sessions: two sessions emphasizing nutrition and two emphasizing exercise; administered on consecutive Saturdays	Group, face-to-face	4	4 weeks	NR
Guilamo-Ramos, 2011[65]	Parent-based	After completing baseline questionnaire, mothers met with a social worker for 30 min and were provided with a packet containing reference materials and family activities to take home and use with child (homework assignments). Packet was a written manual that taught parents effective communication and parenting strategies for reducing adolescent sexual risk behavior. Included nine modules addressing adolescent development and self-esteem, parental self-efficacy to communicate, general parenting strategies, ways to improve the parent-adolescent relationship and communication, adolescent assertiveness skills and techniques for dealing with peer pressure, adolescent sexual behavior, health consequences of sexual risk taking, and birth control and protection. Also included two communication aids. After child completed physician exam, mother met with physician to discuss exam and physician provided a brief endorsement of the Family Talking Together program. Mothers received two booster calls 1 and 5 months after intervention to determine whether they had reviewed the intervention materials and implemented them with their child. Social work interventionist answered any questions the mother had regarding the materials and encouraged the mother to work with the materials.	Individual, face-to-face	3	5 months	Social worker, physician
	Usual care	After completing baseline questionnaire, mother returned to waiting room	NA	NA	NA	NA

Behavioral Counseling to Prevent STIs

Kaiser Permanente Research Affiliates EPC

Appendix C Table 1. Intervention Characteristics of Included Studies Targeting Adolescents

Author, year	Intervention	Description	Delivery and Format Method	No. of Sessions	Duration of Intervention	Provider
Jemmott, 2005[67]	Information-based HIV/STI risk reduction (IG1)	Based on cognitive behavioral theory and previous research with individuals from the study population. Designed to be culturally and developmentally appropriate for inner-city African American and Latino adolescent girls. Information in this intervention group addressed the elevated risk of HIV and STI among inner-city African American and Latino young women, personal vulnerability to HIV and STI, HIV transmission, messages about sex, responsibility for risk reduction in relationships, importance of using condoms, and belief that condoms interfere with sexual enjoyment. HIV educational videotape showed correct condom use. Session lasted 250 min.	Group, face-to-face	1	Once	Bachelors-level facilitator
	Skill-based HIV/STI risk reduction (IG2)	Based on cognitive behavioral theory and previous research with individuals from the study population. Designed to be culturally and developmentally appropriate for inner-city African American and Latino adolescent girls. This intervention addressed beliefs relevant to HIV/STI risk reduction, illustrated correct condom use, and depicted effective condom use negotiation. Participants practiced skills by handling condoms, practicing correct use of condoms with anatomical models, and role playing to increase skill in negotiating the use of condoms. Other issues addressed were the same is in IG1. Session lasted 250 min.	Group, face-to-face	1	Once	Bachelors-level facilitator
	Attention control	Covered beliefs and skills relevant to behaviors associated with the risk of heart disease, cancer, and stroke. Focus on food selection and preparation, physical activity, breast self-examination, cigarette smoking, and alcohol use. Session lasted 250 min.	Group, face-to-face	1	Once	Bachelors-level facilitator

Abbreviations: CG = control group; IG = intervention group; NA = not applicable; NR = not reported; Q&A = question and answer; STI = sexually transmitted infection.

Appendix C Table 2. Intervention Characteristics of Included Studies Targeting Adults or Mixed Ages

Author, year	Intervention	Description	Delivery and Format Method	No. of Sessions	Duration of Intervention	Provider
Berenson, 2012[71]	Contraceptive counseling (IG1)	One-on-one, clinic-based counseling for 45 min delivered by research assistant. Counselor used education and behavioral techniques based on health belief model and geared toward lower health literacy. Components included 1) handouts with instructions for birth control pills and condom use, 2) verbally reviewing instructions using visual aids, 3) developing a cue to assist with adherence to oral contraceptives, 4) discussing pregnancy risk, 5) discussing noncontraceptive beliefs of birth control pills, 6) discussing side effects, 7) discussing STIs and need for condom use, 8) practicing condom application and discussion of condom negotiation skills	Individual, face-to-face	1 session	Once	Experienced research assistants
	Contraceptive counseling plus telephone contact (IG1)	Contraceptive counseling (see above; 45 min); in addition, participants were contacted weekly until they began oral contraception and then monthly for 6 mo by a contraceptive counselor to review correct use, missed doses, side effects, and importance of condom use	Individual, face-to-face and telephone	1 session + 8 calls*	6 mo	Experienced research assistants
	Usual care	Received all contraceptive services from a nurse provider. Participants given oral and written instructions and dispensed 4-mo supply of oral contraception. All participants instructed to initiate contraceptive use within 7 days of starting next menstrual cycle. 24 free condoms provided and a followup appointment made for 3 mo, where additional 9-mo supply of oral contraceptives dispensed	Individual, face-to-face	1 session	Once	Nurse provider
Berkman, 2007[82]	Enhanced SexG	Intervention to decrease episodes of high-risk sex through increased condom use. Decisionmaking skills and strategies to overcome obstacles to condom use presented in relevant and socially appropriate contexts. Participants related exercises to own past and current sexual experiences and rehearsed safer sexual behaviors within and outside the group session. Ten 1-hr sessions held twice a week for 4 weeks, followed by a 4-week break after which the last two sessions held. Session 1: building group cohesion and comfort; Session 2: discuss personal stories, condom use role playing, negotiation skills; Session 3: increase intent to use condoms; Session 4: identify/solve barriers to condom use; Session 5: better response to condom use request by partner; Session 6: increase awareness of UVI/IUAI; Session 7: confidence and ability to have safe sex; Session 8: develop goals; Session 9: reviewing goals and problem solving skills; Session 10: increase goals, commitment, problem solving skills. Booster sessions at 3, 6, and 9 mo after intervention completion to reduce behavioral decay; participants recalled past 3-mo sexual history, brainstormed solutions to risky sexual behaviors. Manualized curriculum. Length of session NR	Group, face-to-face	13 sessions	9 mo	Substance abuse and/or mental health counselors
	Attention control	Money management over 13 sessions, plus one prerandomization HIV prevention session attended by all enrollees in both groups. Length of session NR	Group, face-to-face	13 sessions + 1 HIV prevention session	9 mo	Substance abuse and/or mental health counselors

Appendix C Table 2. Intervention Characteristics of Included Studies Targeting Adults or Mixed Ages

Author, year	Intervention	Description	Delivery and Format Method	No. of Sessions	Duration of Intervention	Provider
Boyer, 1997[88]	Behavioral risk reduction	The 1-hr intervention was designed to increase knowledge about transmission and prevention of STI/HIV; build effective decision-making and communication skills; and identify and modify STI/HIV-related risk factors. Based on a cognitive/behavioral approach that used constructs of the ARRM. Included risk assessment, video, written and verbal information, condoms and anatomical model, and interactive discussion	Individual, face-to-face	4	1 mo	Trained counselor
	Minimal intervention	Standardized risk reduction counseling session (15 min), typically offered to all patients by city clinic counselors at clinic visit	Individual, face-to-face	1	Once	Trained counselor
Carey, 2010[84,157,158]	Brief motivational intervention (IG1)	Based on transtheoretical model, tailored to each patient. Open-ended questions used to understand patient's life circumstances, sexual risk behaviors, and stage-of-change for risk reduction. Counseling appropriate to the patient's stage was delivered; condom use and attendance at intensive intervention emphasized. Session lasted 15 min.	Individual, face-to-face	1	Once	Clinic nurse
	Brief motivational intervention plus intensive informational workshop (IG2)	See IG1 for description of brief motivational intervention (15 min). Participants also invited to workshop (4 hr); they were called until reached to encourage attendance. Intensive informational workshop included information about HIV/STI transmission, prevention, testing, and treatment. Facilitators distributed cards about HIV/STI. Participants took turns reading statements aloud and discussed statements. Participants placed cards labeled with different sexual activities along a risk continuum. Workshop concluded with a Q&A game show covering workshop content	Individual and group, face-to-face	2	Once	Clinic nurse, workshop facilitators
	Brief motivational intervention plus intensive motivation behavioral skills workshop (IG3)	See IG1 for description of brief motivational intervention. Participants also invited to workshop (4 hr); they were called until reached to encourage attendance. Workshop included three components: information, motivation, and behavioral skills. Information: HIV transmission and prevention information. Motivation: received local HIV/STI rates; watched a video of infected HIV individuals and discussed what it would be like; placed sexual behaviors along a risk continuum, discussed basis for each appraisal, and reflected on own sexual behaviors. Behavior skills: engaged in interactive exercises to learn personal triggers for risky sex, strategies for managing triggers, talk with partner about condom use and safer sexual behaviors, apply condom; role playing allowed practice of skills. Workshop concluded with goal setting and a review	Individual and group, face-to-face	2	Once	Clinic nurse, workshop facilitators
	Brief information plus intensive informational workshop (IG4)	See CG for brief information intervention. See IG2 for intensive information workshop. Same characteristics as IG2 or IG3.	Individual and group, face-to-face	2	Once	Clinic nurse, workshop facilitators

Appendix C Table 2. Intervention Characteristics of Included Studies Targeting Adults or Mixed Ages

Author, year	Intervention	Description	Delivery and Format Method	No. of Sessions	Duration of Intervention	Provider
	Brief information plus intensive motivation behavior skills workshop (IG5)	See CG for brief information intervention. See IG3 for intensive information motivation behavioral skills workshop. Same characteristics as IG2 or IG3.	Individual and group, face-to-face	2	Once	Clinic nurse, workshop facilitators
	Minimal intervention	Brief information intervention delivered via DVD in a private room. DVD content adapted from a validated intervention and included information about HIV/STIs, testing; sexual risk reduction options presented in an engaging and culturally appropriate style (15 min). DVD also stated attending educational and safer sex workshops could help people stay healthy. Nurse met briefly with patients and asked a series of close-ended questions to assess sexual risk behavior and stage-of-change for risk reduction. Participants were not invited to workshop	Individual, face-to-face	1	Once	Clinic nurse
Carey, 2004[64]	HIV risk reduction	Sought to enhance participant's knowledge, motivation, and behavioral skills about risky sexual behavior. Sessions included information (sexual behavior, HIV/STIs) and motivational components; value of HIV testing and counseling; motivational exercises to increase risk awareness and desensitization, encourage identification of pros/cons of risk reduction strategies, discuss social norms regarding risk and safer sex and encourage mutual social support for risk reduction; developed safer sex, self-management, condom negotiation and sexual assertiveness skills; prepare participants to obtain, store, and use condoms correctly (IMB model); develop coping strategies and self-efficacy for dealing with high-risk situations. Included homework and interactive role playing. Length of session NR	Group, face-to-face	10	5 weeks	Masters and doctoral level facilitators
	Attention control (CG1)	Sought to enhance participants knowledge, motivation, and behavioral skills about risky substance use behavior. Used SCT framework to promote responsible substance use; used interactive role play exercises and motivational interventions. Sessions included knowledge, motivation, and self-management skills to reduce caffeine use; preventing, reducing, or eliminating tobacco use and harmful alcohol consumption; and solidification of long-term substance use behavior change goals. Included homework. Length of session NR	Group, face-to-face	10	5 weeks	Masters and doctoral level facilitators
	Usual care (CG2)	Standard outpatient psychiatric care including medication, psychotherapy, and case management services. No prohibition regarding the discussion of HIV or substance use. Length of session NR.	NR	1	Once	NR

Appendix C Table 2. Intervention Characteristics of Included Studies Targeting Adults or Mixed Ages

Author, year	Intervention	Description	Delivery and Format Method	No. of Sessions	Duration of Intervention	Provider
Cianelli, 2012[75]	Mano a Mano-Mujer HIV prevention	Based on social cognitive model of behavioral change, contextual tailoring, and WHO primary health care model. Six 2-hr sessions delivered in small groups with an average of 8 to 10 women. Sessions covered HIV/AIDS in the community and Chile, STIs, prevention of HIV/AIDS (abstinence, mutual fidelity, condom use), negotiation and communication with a partner, prevention and control of domestic violence, substance abuse, and importance of family. Sessions included role play; participatory sessions, videos, and discussions used to build self-efficacy and communication skills. Intervention took place in community settings.	Group, face-to-face	6	NR	Trained health educator
	Waitlist	Delayed intervention	NA	NA	NA	NA
Cortes-Borday, 2010[86]	Counseling plus educational leaflet	Educational leaflet created by group of experts, based on best available evidence, with objective of helping patients to understand HPV infection and prevent risk behavior. Leaflet titled "What should you know about condylomas or genital warts?" included clear, short answers to 10 simple questions related to acquisition of disease, clinical features, treatment, assessment of sex partners, pregnancy, malignant change, and use of condoms; key points for prevention of STIs. Gynecologist discussed items in leaflet. Length of session NR	Individual, face-to-face	1	Once	Gynecologist
	Usual care	Noncounseling, no leaflet. Length of session NR	Individual, face-to-face	1	Once	Gynecologist
Crosby, 2009[87]	Focus on the Future	Predicated on the IMB model. Men learned about variety of condoms, water-based lubricant better than oil-based (oil-based can deteriorate condom); encouraged to feel good about using condoms, that they are compatible with sexual pleasure, and that they protect them from acquiring STIs. Men allowed to respond to HIV/AIDS burden posters in which advisor responded to questions, problems, and concerns regarding safer sex with female partners. Men prompted to think about ways to initiate condom use and skill acquisition (demonstration of correct condom use and lubricant application). Men encouraged to use condoms that fit well and provided a sense of security. Men provided with water-based lubricants and 12+ condoms of any brand and size. Also received nurse-delivered messages on condom use per CDC guidelines (few minutes) informing them that condoms are effective at preventing STIs and additional 12+ condoms of one particular size and brand. 45- to 50-minute session.	Individual, face-to-face	1	Once	Lay health advisors
	Minimal intervention	Received nurse-delivered messages for a few minutes on condom use per CDC guidelines informing them that condoms are effective at preventing STIs and additional 12+ condoms of one particular size and brand.	Individual, face-to-face	1	Once	Nurse

Appendix C Table 2. Intervention Characteristics of Included Studies Targeting Adults or Mixed Ages

Author, year	Intervention	Description	Delivery and Format Method	No. of Sessions	Duration of Intervention	Provider
Ehrhardt, 2002[81,105,163-166]	8-session sex-specific HIV/STI risk reduction (IG1)	Based on the ARRM and designed to decrease unsafe sexual practices in women. Each group session lasted 2 hr; one topic covered per session. Topics included caring about getting HIV/STIs, avoiding partners who don't care, best ways to protect self, resources to find out if infected, ways to ask and influence partner to use protection, ways to refuse sex/unprotected sex, and ways to continue protecting self and others. Group activities included role playing, problem solving, letter writing, attitude confrontation, storytelling, and modeling. A 2-hr booster session was provided 9 mo after baseline to review progress, take pride in achievements, receive assistance, help other group members, and be renewed by the group's support (Miller 2000). Female condoms were provided and discussed in a session and made available to participants in future sessions if desired (Hoffman 2003)	Group, face-to-face	8	8 weeks	Facilitators
	4-session sex-specific HIV/STI risk reduction (IG2)	Based on the ARRM and designed to decrease unsafe sexual practices in women. Each group session lasted 2 hr; two topics covered per session. Topics included caring about getting HIV/STIs, avoiding partners who don't care, best ways to protect self, resources to find out if infected, ways to ask and influence partner to use protection, ways to refuse sex/unprotected sex, and ways to continue protecting self and others. To make this version of the intervention as similar as possible to the 8-session one, the same topic areas were covered and less time was spent on group exercises. Group activities included role playing, problem solving, letter writing, attitude confrontation, storytelling, and modeling. Female condoms were provided and discussed in a session and made available to participants in future sessions if desired (Hoffman 2003)	Group, face-to-face	4	4 weeks	Facilitators
	Minimal intervention	Risk assessment only	Individual, NR	NR	NR	NR
Jemmott, 2007[79,160]	Group skills HIV/STI risk reduction (IG1)	Based on social cognitive theory. 200-minute session with 3 to 5 participants. Designed to increase skills regarding condom use, to allay participants concerns about the adverse effects of condom use on sexual enjoyment, group discussions, brainstorming, videos, interactive exercises, games, condom demonstrations, practice and role playing to increase self-efficacy and skills related to correct use of condoms and negotiation of condom use with sexual partners	Group, face-to-face	1	Once	Trained nurses
	Group informational HIV/STI risk reduction (IG2)	Based on social cognitive theory, 200-min session with 3 to 5 participants. Designed to increase perception of vulnerability to HIV/STIs, increase knowledge about transmission and prevention of HIV/STIs. Involved group discussions, brainstorming, videos, interactive exercises, and games. Did not provide behavioral skill demonstrations, practice, or address participants' beliefs about adverse effects of condom use on sexual enjoyment.	Group, face-to-face	1	Once	Trained nurses

Appendix C Table 2. Intervention Characteristics of Included Studies Targeting Adults or Mixed Ages

Author, year	Intervention	Description	Delivery and Format Method	No. of Sessions	Duration of Intervention	Provider
	Individual skills HIV/STI risk reduction (IG3)	Based on social cognitive theory, 20-min session tailored to the specific needs of each participant. Designed to increase skills for condom use; review of HIV/STI brochure, video clips, condom demonstration, practice, and role playing to increase self-efficacy and skill related to correct condom use and negotiation of condom use with partner	Individual, face-to-face	1	Once	Trained nurses
	Individual informational HIV/STI risk reduction (IG4)	Based on social cognitive theory, 20-min session tailored to the specific needs of each participant. Designed to increase knowledge about HIV/STI transmission, prevention, and personal vulnerability; reviewed HIV/STI prevention brochure and discussion of basic HIV/STI risk reduction information. No behavioral skill demonstrations or practice	Individual, face-to-face	1	Once	Trained nurses
	Attention control	General health promotion focused on diet, physical exercise, alcohol and tobacco use associated with risk of heart disease, stroke and cancer; not focused on HIV/STI risk behaviors. Length of session NR	NR	NR	NR	Trained nurses
Kamb, 1998[58,144-147]	Enhanced counseling (IG1)	Encouraged consistent condom use for vaginal and anal sex with all partners; tailored to each's personal risks, included HIV test. Four sessions based on social cognitive and reasoned action theories sought to change key theoretical elements to condom use (attitudes). Session 1 (20 min); Sessions 2-4 (60 min). Test results provided during Session 3. First 3 sessions concluded with behavioral goal setting exercises to arrive at a small behavioral risk reduction step before next session. Last session developed a longer-term, risk reduction plan.	Individual, face-to-face	4	4 weeks	Counselor
	Brief counseling (IG2)	Encouraged consistent condom use for vaginal and anal sex with all partners; tailored to each's personal risks, included HIV test. Two sessions modeled after CDC HIV counseling for patients attending public clinics and HIV test site guidelines. Both sessions 20 min. Session 1 concluded with behavioral goal setting exercise. Session 2 included HIV test results and discussion and review of behavioral goal and developed a longer-term risk reduction plan. Objective included assess actual and self-perceived HIV/STI risk, recognize barriers to risk reduction, negotiate acceptable and achievable risk reduction plan, and support patient-initiated behavior change.	Individual, face-to-face	2	10 days	Counselor
	Minimal intervention plus followup visits (CG1)	Encouraged consistent condom use for vaginal and anal sex with all partners; tailored to each's personal risks, included HIV test. Two informational sessions with brief messages about HIV/STI prevention. Session 1 (5 min) conducted by treating physician, Session 2 (5 min) informed of HIV test results and didactic prevention messages.	Individual, face-to-face	2	10 days	Physician

Appendix C Table 2. Intervention Characteristics of Included Studies Targeting Adults or Mixed Ages

Author, year	Intervention	Description	Delivery and Format Method	No. of Sessions	Duration of Intervention	Provider
	Minimal intervention (CG2)	Encouraged consistent condom use for vaginal and anal sex with all partners; tailored to each's personal risks, included HIV test. Two informational sessions with brief messages about HIV/STI prevention. Session 1 (5 min) conducted by treating physician, Session 2 (5 min) informed of HIV test results and didactic prevention messages. No followup visits.	Individual, face-to-face	2	10 days	Physician
Kershaw, 2009[59]	Centering Pregnancy Plus	Prenatal care within a group setting, curriculum provided by a trained practitioner. 10 sessions (2 hr each) during pregnancy cover self-care activities such as weight and blood pressure assessment, group discussion to address prenatal care, childbirth preparation, and postpartum care. Included 3 sessions (sessions 4, 5, 7) where 40 min were devoted to HIV prevention skills; based on social cognitive theory and the ecological model. Session 4, participants watched testimonials of HIV+ adolescents, discussed barriers and benefits to condom use, personalized HIV/STI risk, set safe sex behavior goals. Session 5, developed sex partner communication skills through role playing and modeling. Session 7, reinforced communication skills through role play and modeling, evaluated goals and set new goals for safe sexual behavior after pregnancy.	Group, face-to-face	10	NR	Trained practitioner (midwife or obstetrician)
	Attention control (CG1)	Prenatal care within a group setting, curriculum provided by a trained practitioner. 10 sessions (2 hr each) during pregnancy cover self-care activities such as weight and blood pressure assessment, group discussion to address prenatal care, childbirth preparation, and postpartum care. No HIV-specific content or skill building.	Group, face-to-face	10	NR	Trained practitioner (midwife or obstetrician)
	Usual care (CG2)	Consistent prenatal care.	NR, face-to-face	10	NR	Trained practitioner (midwife or obstetrician)
Marion, 2009[85]	Well Woman program	Based on the interaction model of client health behavior. Includes individualized and group sessions along with comprehensive care management delivered by nurse practitioners (NPs). Culturally specific, personalized, goal-oriented counseling and peer-led group classes that integrated individually tailored and group-targeted STI diagnosis, treatment, and preventive services over the study period. Conducted in 2 phases. Intensive (first 2 mo) phase: participants met with NP for a complete medical and sexual history, physical exam, and individualized counseling focused on building knowledge, skill, and will related to STI prevention practices (having 1 sex partner, negotiating condom use, adhering to STI treatment); attend 2 peer educator-led group sessions (STI knowledge, skill, and will building); additional meeting with NP for individualized counseling. Maintenance phase (3-12 mo): single group sessions during mo 4 and 8; met with NP for individualized counseling during mo 6 and 12. Free male and female condoms and lubricants were distributed at all individual and group sessions. Length of sessions 5-7 hr.	Individual and group, face-to-face	8	12 mo	Nurse practitioners and peer educator

Appendix C Table 2. Intervention Characteristics of Included Studies Targeting Adults or Mixed Ages

Author, year	Intervention	Description	Delivery and Format Method	No. of Sessions	Duration of Intervention	Provider
	Minimal intervention	Included a 10 to 20 min educational session, STI testing, and directions to seek usual care. 10-min standardized STI presentations, STI care continued with community providers. Conducted in a research lab. At study completion, received a condensed set of the STI prevention intervention components.	Individual, face-to-face	4	NR	Research associate
Marrazzo, 2011[74,161,162]	Motivational interviewing	Patients instructed on how to use behaviors aimed at reducing likelihood of transferring vaginal fluid to female partners during sex and provided safe sex kits (male condoms, nitrile gloves, water-based lubrication). Behaviors targeted included use of gloves during digital-vaginal sex, use of condom if insertion toys were shared, and use of lubricant provided or another water-based lubricant. Treated with vaginal metronidazole. Length of session NR.	Individual, face-to-face	1	Once	Study staff
	Attention control	Patients received information on the need for adherence to routine Pap smear screening guidelines. Did not receive information on sexual behavior modification or the safe sex kit. Treated with vaginal metronidazole. Length of session NR.	Individual, face-to-face	1	Once	Study staff
Metsch, 2013[90]	HIV testing and risk reduction counseling	Risk reduction counseling included discussion of patient's specific HIV/STI risk behaviors and negotiation of achievable risk reduction steps; may have included unprotected sex with multiple partners, increased sexual risk taking due to heavy substance use, lack of discussion of HIV status with sexual partners. A concrete, realistic risk reduction plan was developed. Also explained rapid HIV testing process, including window period and interpretation of test findings. Nonreactive tests: counselor repeated test information, reviewed risk reduction plan, and offered referrals, lubricant, and condoms. Reactive test results: posttesting counseling about test results and the need to avoid behaviors that pose a transmission risk. Patients with confirmed results were linked to HIV primary care. Median of 28 min for counseling, 7 min for results.	Individual, face-to-face	1	Once	Counselor
	Minimal intervention	Rapid HIV test and verbal information about HIV per CDC recommendations; provided with the test kit patient information pamphlet. Nonreactive tests: counselor repeated test information. Reactive test: posttesting counseling about test results and the need to avoid behaviors that pose a transmission risk. Median of 3 min for information, 3 min for results.	Individual, face-to-face	1	Once	Counselor
Neumann, 2011[80]	VOICES/ VOCES HIV/STI prevention	45-min intervention intended to increase STI knowledge, proper condom use, and condom negotiation skills. Facilitator delivers in a private room with 4 to 8 participants. Information on STI/HIV risk behaviors and condom use delivered with culturally specific videos, group discussion, poster of various condom brand features; role playing of condom negotiation modeled in videos and provided with free condom samples.	Group, face-to-face and video	1	Once	Facilitator
	Usual care	Regular clinic services, received free condoms and coupons.	NA	NA	NA	NA

Appendix C Table 2. Intervention Characteristics of Included Studies Targeting Adults or Mixed Ages

Author, year	Intervention	Description	Delivery and Format Method	No. of Sessions	Duration of Intervention	Provider
Peipert, 2008[72,159]	Tailored TTM expert system	Model conceptualizes a progression through stages of change toward consistent dual condom and contraceptive use through pre-contemplation, contemplation, preparation, action, and maintenance. Multimedia expert system administers questions on screen and by voice, includes pictures and music. Responses used by expert system for treatment feedback based on participants' readiness to change behavior. Feedback written at 6th grade level to ensure comprehension. Three sessions: baseline, 1 mo, and 2 mo. Content divided into 1) current stage of change, 2) pros/cons of condom and other contraceptive use, 3) help with at-risk situations and appropriate coping responses to increase efficacy for condom and other contraceptive behavior, 4) information about over- and under-use of those processes appropriate for that individual's stage of change, 5) more tips and strategies to facilitate progress. Length of session NR.	Individual, computer-based	3	80 days	NA
	Minimal intervention	Standard contraceptive and STI prevention intervention chosen by patient. Information included benefits of dual and individual method use, risk appraisal for STI/HIV, places to obtain condoms, tips for using condoms correctly, risks and benefits of hormonal contraceptives, side effect information and ways of dealing with side effects, and effectiveness data for all contraceptive methods. Also received advice to use condoms to prevent diseases and an additional method of contraception to prevent pregnancy in addition to being provided with educational pamphlets (nontailored). Length of session NR.	Individual, computer-based	1	Once	NA
Petersen, 2007[70]	STI risk reduction	Adapted from motivational interviewing; emphasized three elements: exploring discrepancies between pregnancy intention and contraceptive use; between STI risk and condom use; sharing information with participants and promoting behaviors to reduce risk. Initial session encouraged women to adopt consistent, effective contraceptive and condom use to prevent STIs. Counseling individualized to current contraceptive use and risk reduction. Obtainment or referral for any type of contraception available. In-person or telephone booster session focused on progress on risk reduction steps 2 mo after initial session. Length of session NR.	Individual, face-to-face and telephone	2	2 mo	Trained health educator
	Attention control	Brief general counseling on prevention health care (smoking, diet, exercise), excluded STI and pregnancy prevention; no further counseling. Length of session NR.	Individual, face-to-face	1	NR	Trained health educator
Proude, 2004[76]	Safe sex	Brief behavioral advice based on brief risk assessment (risk for STIs, unwanted pregnancy, and hepatitis B or C) and resources, including condoms and lubricant, educational pamphlets on condom use, STIs/HIV, hepatitis B (including vaccination), alcohol and drug information services.	Individual, face-to-face	1	Once	Family physician
	Attention control	Tobacco screening and counseling. Length of session NR.	Individual, face-to-face	1	Once	Family physician

Appendix C Table 2. Intervention Characteristics of Included Studies Targeting Adults or Mixed Ages

Author, year	Intervention	Description	Delivery and Format Method	No. of Sessions	Duration of Intervention	Provider
Scholes, 2003[83]	Self-help mailings	Tailored 12-page self-help magazine style booklet; safe sex kit containing male and female condoms, condom carrying case, and instructions on condom use. After 3 mo, tailored booster feedback newsletter and condom packet.	Individual, mailings	2	3 mo	NA
	Usual care	NR	NR	NR	NR	NR
Shain, 1999[57,154-156]	Behavioral cognitive risk reduction	Based on ARRM. Session 1 focused on recognition of risk (increase awareness, address myths, address belief that disease is "dirty" and encourage acceptance of responsibility for infection, discuss selection of sex partners, provide information about STIs, increase awareness of personal risk), session 2 focused on commitment to change (provide information about STIs and early treatment, teach what to ask partners about current behavior and history, teach use of condoms with models, barriers to condom use, discuss what women want from a relationship, teach decisionmaking skills), and session 3 focused on acquisition of skills (increase skills for communicating and negotiating, teach basic skills to deal with sexual dysfunction resulting from condom use, raise feelings of self-efficacy, more practice of condom application, identify and discuss triggers to unsafe sex, set goals, facilitate bonding and mutual support, encourage sharing of information with others). Included videotape, props for skill building exercises, graphic materials designed for low-literacy groups, and role play. Sessions were each 3 to 4 hr.	Group, face-to-face	3	3 weeks	Trained facilitators
Shain, 2004[73,167]	Minimal intervention	Individualized counseling (15 min) according to the patient's sexual history and her responses to a test of knowledge.	Individual, face-to-face	1	Once	Nurse clinician
	Standard behavioral cognitive counseling (IG1)	Interactive STI counseling (individual) and standard behavioral cognitive intervention (group). Three weekly small-group sessions lasting approximately 3 hr; separate sessions for each ethnic group with ethnically-matched female facilitators. Adapted ARRM for target population. Overall goals to have women recognize STI risk, commit to behavior change, acquire necessary skills to effect change, and be vigilant in promptly seeking care for possible infection.	Individual and group, face-to-face	4	3 weeks	Facilitators
	Standard behavioral cognitive counseling plus support groups (IG2)	Interactive STI counseling (individual) and standard behavioral cognitive intervention (group). Three weekly small-group sessions lasting approximately 3 hr; separate sessions held for each ethnic group with ethnically-matched female facilitators. Adapted ARRM for target population. Overall goals to have women recognize STI risk, commit to behavior change, acquire necessary skills to effect change, and be vigilant in promptly seeking care for possible infection. Optional enhanced support group sessions including discussion of changing behavior, abuse, social/sexual roles, love, trust, and intimacy lasting 90 min.	Individual and group, face-to-face	9	5 mo	Facilitators

Appendix C Table 2. Intervention Characteristics of Included Studies Targeting Adults or Mixed Ages

Author, year	Intervention	Description	Delivery and Format Method	No. of Sessions	Duration of Intervention	Provider
	Minimal intervention	15- to 20-min interactive counseling emphasizing full treatment of participant and partners, avoidance of sexual activity until treatment completed, mutual monogamy, taking time between partners to be selective, consistent and correct condom use, avoidance of douching, and seeking care whenever they suspected infection. Participants informed intervention would be available to them after study completion.	Individual, face-to-face	1	Once	NR
Warner, 2006[78]	Safe in the City video	Based on integrated theoretical approach to achieving health behavior change. "Safe in the City" video (23 min) incorporated key prevention messages aimed at increasing knowledge and perception of STI/HIV risk, promoting positive attitudes toward condom use, and building self-efficacy and skills to facilitate partner treatment, safer sex, and the acquisition, negotiation, and use of condoms. Video contained vignettes that modeled young couples of various races/ethnicities and sexual orientations negotiating safer sex. Animated segments demonstrated proper condom use and variety of available condoms. Posters in waiting and exam room directed attention to the video and reinforced key messages. Condoms and educational pamphlets on STI prevention available to all patients.	Individual, video	1	Once	NA
	Usual care	Standard waiting room experience, absence of video and posters; may have included television programming, music, or both (varied by site). Condoms and educational pamphlets on STI prevention available to all patients.	NA	NA	NA	NA
Wenger, 1992[7]	HIV/AIDS education (IG1)	Education module consisted of a multimedia presentation in a small group format led by physicians familiar with HIV counseling. Module lasted 1 hr and consisted of a videotape (11 min), lecture (15 min), role play (15 min), discussion (15 min), and distribution of written material. Scripted lecture covered AIDS introduction, routes of transmission and safe sex behaviors, obstacles to using condoms and communicating with partner about HIV risk factors, role of substances in unsafe sex, instruction on condom use, and information on HIV testing. Encouraged study participation, allowed for questions, and concluded with lively discussion. Offered a list of locations where a free, anonymous HIV test could be obtained.	Group, face-to-face	1	Once	Physician
	HIV/AIDS education plus testing (IG2)	Same as above, plus subjects received an HIV antibody test. Results were given to subjects approximately 1 week after blood draw, in person or by telephone, accompanied by the same risk reduction message given during the educational module; no individualized posttest counseling was given.	Group, face-to-face	1	Once	Physician
	Usual care	No further participation in the study until completion of followup questionnaire. Offered a list of locations where a free, anonymous HIV antibody test could be obtained.	Individual, NR	NR	NR	NR

Appendix C Table 2. Intervention Characteristics of Included Studies Targeting Adults or Mixed Ages

Author, year	Intervention	Description	Delivery and Format Method	No. of Sessions	Duration of Intervention	Provider
Wingood 2013[89] Good	HIV prevention intervention	Intervention (4 hr) informed by CDC HIV guidelines and social cognitive theory informed content by seeking to enhance participants' attitudes and skills in abstaining from sexual intercourse, practicing low-risk sexual behaviors, avoiding untreated STIs, using condoms consistently, and refraining from having multiple and concurrent sex partners. Content emphasized valuing one's body, perceiving one's body as a temple (culturally appropriate), information on risk of STI/HIV when engaging in concurrency, and discussing partner selection strategies that encouraged monogamy. Also informed by theory of gender and power to enhance women's awareness of power imbalances and increasing self-sufficiency, educating participants about gender-related HIV prevention strategies.	Group, face-to-face	2	2 weeks	Trained health educators
	Attention control	Emphasized nutrition education (4 hr).	Group, face-to-face	1	Once	Trained health educators

*Estimated.

Abbreviations: ARRM = AIDS Risk Reduction Model; CDC = Centers for Disease Control and Prevention; CG = control group; IG = intervention group; IMB = information, motivation, and behavioral; MI = motivational interviewing; min = minute(s); NA = not applicable; NP = nurse practitioner; NR = not reported; STI = sexually transmitted infection; Q&A = question and answer; SCT = social cognitive theory; TTM = transtheoretical model; UVI = unprotected vaginal intercourse; UAI = unprotected anal intercourse.

Appendix C Table 3. Results From Included Studies Targeting Adolescents—STIs

Author, year Quality	Setting	Risk	N rand	Population (mean age, y)	STI History	Outcome, ascertainment	F/U (mo)	IG Results	CG Results	Between Group Difference: Point Estimate (95% CI) or P-value
Low-intensity (<30 min)										
Boekeloo, 1999[63,143] Fair	Washington DC, primary care	Low/mix	219	Adolescents ages 12 to 15 y (NR)	Treated for STI: 5.9%	% treated for an STI (NR), self-reported (since previous assessment)	BL 3 9	7.5 2.2 1.1	4.5 4.7 5.8	NSD NSD NSD
Moderate-intensity (30 to 120 min)										
Kershaw, 2009[59] Fair	Atlanta, GA, and New Haven, CT, primary care	Increased	513 (sub-group)	Pregnant adolescents age <20 y (NR)	Lifetime STI: "more than half"	% STI (chlamydia, gonorrhea), laboratory	12	9.3	CG1: 12.6 CG2: 20.3	IG vs. CG1: OR, 0.67 (0.30 to 1.45) IG vs. CG2: OR, 0.37 (0.17 to 0.77)
Kamb (mod IG), 1998[58,144-147] Fair	5 US cities, STI clinic	Increased	508 (sub-group)	Sexually active adolescents ages 14 to 19 y (NR)	BL STI: 32%*	% STI (chlamydia, gonorrhea, syphilis, HIV), laboratory	12	IG2: 17.5	26.6	IG2 vs. CG: adjusted OR, 0.53 (0.32 to 0.86)
High-intensity (>120 min)										
Jemmott, 2005[67] Fair	Philadelphia, PA, primary care	Increased	682	Sexually active African American or Latino adolescent girls ages 12 to 19 y (15.5)	BL STI: 21.6%	% STI (gonorrhea, chlamydia, trichomoniasis), laboratory	BL 6 12	IG1: 26 IG2: 22.8 IG1: 15.5 IG2: 15.8 IG1: 15.4 IG2: 10.5	16.9 14.8 18.2	NSD IG1 vs. CG: p=0.89 IG2 vs. CG: p=0.80 IG1 vs. CG: p=0.44 IG2 vs. CG: p=0.05
DiClemente, 2004[68,148-153] Good	Birmingham, AL, primary care	Increased	522	Sexually active African American adolescent girls ages 14 to 18 y (16)	BL STI: G: 5.2% C: 17.4% T: 12.6%	Gonorrhea, unadjusted rate per 100 person-mo, laboratory	12	0.9	0.7	Adjusted OR, 0.14 (0.01 to 3.02)
						Chlamydia, unadjusted rate per 100 person-mo, laboratory	12	2.1	2.0	Adjusted OR, 0.17 (0.03 to 0.92)
						Trichomoniasis, unadjusted rate per 100 person-mo, laboratory	12	0.9	1.2	Adjusted OR, 0.37 (0.09 to 1.46)
Kamb (high IG), 1998[58,144-147] Fair	5 US cities, STI clinic	Increased	512 (sub-group)	Sexually active adolescents ages 14 to 19 y (NR)	BL STI: 32%*	% STI (chlamydia, gonorrhea, syphilis, HIV), laboratory	12	IG1: 17.2	26.6	IG1 vs. CG: adjusted OR, 0.54 (0.33 to 0.88)
Champion, 2012[69] Fair	Southwestern US, research clinic	Prior STI	559	Ethnic minority adolescent girls with STI or abuse (16.5)	Lifetime STI: 100% (of analyzed sample)	% new STI (gonorrhea, chlamydia), laboratory	6 12	0 4.8	6.6 13.2	p=0.001 Adjusted OR, 0.035 (0.002 to 0.53)
Shain, 1999[57,154-156] Fair	San Antonio, TX, research clinic	Prior STI	148 (sub-group)	Adolescent Mexican American and African American girls ages 14 to 18 y with a nonviral STI (NR)	BL STI: 100%	% STI (chlamydia, gonorrhea), laboratory	6 12	12.1 24.2	25.6 40.2	OR, 2.50 (1.03 to 6.08); p=0.04 OR, 2.11 (1.03 to 4.3); p=0.04

*Data for entire study population, which included adults and adolescents.

Abbreviations: BL = baseline; C = chlamydia; CG = control group; CI = confidence interval; F/U = followup; G = gonorrhea; HIV = human immunodeficiency virus; IG = intervention group; NR = not reported; NSD = no significant difference; OR = odds ratio; rand = randomized; STI = sexually transmitted infection; T = trichomoniasis.

Appendix C Table 4. Results From Included Studies Targeting Adults—STIs

Author, year Quality	Setting	Risk	N rand	Population (mean age, y)	STI History	Outcome, ascertainment	F/U (mo)	IG Results	CG Results	Between Group Difference: Point Estimate (95% CI) or P-value
Low-intensity (<30 min)										
Scholes, 2003[83] Fair	WA and NC, primary care	General	1210	Sexually active nonmonogamous women ages 18 to 24 y (21)	Lifetime STI: 27%	% STI (NR), self-reported	6	3.5	3.6	Adjusted OR, 0.97 (0.48 to 1.96)
Carey (low IG), 2010[84,157,158] Fair	Syracuse, NY, STI clinic	Increased	496	Adults age ≥18 y with high-risk behavior in past 3 mo (29.2)	BL STI: 18.1%	% new STI (gonorrhea, chlamydia, HIV), laboratory (since previous assessment)	3 6 12	NR NR NR	NR NR NR	NSD NSD NSD
Peipert, 2008[72,159] Fair	Providence, RI, primary care and Planned Parenthood	Increased	542	Women ages 13 to 35 y at high risk for STI or unplanned pregnancy due to age, behavior, history of STI or pregnancy (median, 22)	Lifetime STI: 47%	% STI (chlamydia, gonorrhea, trichomoniasis, syphilis, HIV), laboratory	24	16	16	Adjusted HR, 1.4 (0.76 to 2.58)
Warner, 2008[78] Good	Denver, CO, Long Beach, CA, and San Francisco, CA, STI clinic	Increased	40,282	All patients (NR)	BL STI: 15.5%	% ≥1 STI (gonorrhea, chlamydia, trichomoniasis, syphilis, HIV, laboratory	14.8	4.9	5.7	Adjusted HR, 0.91 (0.84 to 0.99)
Jemmott (low IG), 2007[79,160] Good	Newark, NJ, primary care	Increased	322	African American women ages 18 to 45 y (27.2)	BL STI: 20.3%	% STI (gonorrhea, chlamydia, trichomoniasis), laboratory	6 12	IG3: 0.22 IG4: 0.17 IG3: 0.14 IG4: 0.22	0.15 0.27	IG1/IG3 vs. CG: p=0.35 IG1/IG3 vs. IG2/IG4: p=0.38 IG1/IG3 vs. CG: p=0.03 IG1/IG3 vs. IG2/IG4: p=0.13
Marrazzo, 2011[74,161,162] Fair	Seattle, WA, research clinic	Prior STI	89	Women ages 16 to 30 y with BV who have sex with women (25.4)	Current BV: 100%	Bacterial vaginosis, incident episodes per 100 person-mo, laboratory and clinic exam	3	9.2	7.7	Adjusted HR, 1.03 (0.54 to 1.97)
Moderate-intensity (30 to 120 min)										
Petersen, 2007[70] Fair	Chapel Hill, NC, primary care	General	764	Women ages 16 to 44 y at risk for unintended pregnancy (no IUD or sterilization) (NR)	NR	% STI (chlamydia, "other"), medical chart review	12	NR	NR	NSD
Metsch, 2013[90] Good	7 states and Washington, DC, STI clinics	Increased	5012	Adults age ≥18 y seeking services at an STI clinic (NR)	BL STI: 44.3%	% STI (syphilis, HSV-2, HIV, gonorrhea, chlamydia, trichomoniasis), laboratory	6	12.3	11.1	Adjusted risk ratio, 1.12 (1.94 to 1.33)
Berenson (mod IG), 2012[71] Fair	Southeast TX, reproductive health clinic	Increased	771	Sexually active women ages 16 to 24 y (19.9)	Lifetime: 26.1%	% participants with ≥1 STI (NR), self-reported or medical record review	12	IG1: 3.1	4.6	IG1 vs. CG: HR, 1.01 (0.46 to 2.21)
Neumann, 2011[80] Fair	Harlem, NY, and Puerto Rico, STI clinics	Increased	3365	Adults age ≥18 y, 99% racial/ethnic minority (29.3)	BL STI: 22.2%	% STI (chancroid, chlamydia, gonorrhea, granuloma inguinale, lymphogranuloma venereum, nongonococcal urethritis, mucopurulent cervicitis, syphilis, HIV, herpes), laboratory	22	10.1	13.5	Adjusted HR, 0.78 (0.64 to 0.96)
Kershaw, 2009[59] Fair	Atlanta, GA, and New Haven, CT, primary care	Increased	534 (subgroup)	Pregnant women age ≥20 y (NR)	Lifetime STI: "more than half"	% STI (chlamydia, gonorrhea), laboratory	12	10.5	CG1: 7.6 CG2: 7.5	NSD

Appendix C Table 4. Results From Included Studies Targeting Adults—STIs

Author, year Quality	Setting	Risk	N rand	Population (mean age, y)	STI History	Outcome, ascertainment	F/U (mo)	IG Results	CG Results	Between Group Difference: Point Estimate (95% CI) or P-value
Kamb (mod IG) 1998[58,144-147] Fair	5 US cities, STI clinic	Increased	2382 (subgroup)	Adults age ≥20 y (NR)	BL STI: 32%*	% STI (chlamydia, gonorrhea, syphilis, HIV), laboratory	12	IG2: 10.8	12.0	Age 20–25 y: IG2 vs. CG: 0.91 (0.62 to 1.3) Age >25 y: IG2 vs. CG: 0.78 (0.53 to 1.13)
Crosby, 2009[87] Fair	Southern US, STI clinic	Prior STI	266	African American men ages 18 to 29 y with newly diagnosed STI and recent experience with condoms (23.2)	BL STI: 100%	% STI reinfection (NR, includes chlamydia, gonorrhea), medical record review	6	31.9	50.4	Adjusted OR, 0.32 (0.12 to 0.86)
High-intensity (>120 min)										
Wingood, 2013[89] Fair	Atlanta, GA, HMO	Increased	848	Sexually active African American women ages 18 to 29 y (22.0)	BL STI: 17%	% STI (any nonviral: chlamydia, gonorrhea, trichomoniasis), laboratory	6 12	6.1 9.5	9.7 12.0	Adjusted OR, 0.52 (0.26 to 1.04) Adjusted OR, 0.67 (0.37 to 1.20) GEE adjusted OR, 0.62 (0.40 to 0.96)
Berenson (high IG), 2012[71] Good	Southeast TX, reproductive health clinic	Increased	772	Sexually active women ages 16 to 24 y (19.9)	Lifetime: 26.1%	% participants with ≥1 STI (NR, self-reported or medical record review)	12	IG2: 3.4	4.6	IG2 vs. CG: HR, 0.70 (0.31 to 1.59)
Carey (high IG) 2010[84,157,158] Fair	Syracuse, NY, STI clinic	Increased	1235	Adults age ≥18 y with high-risk behavior in past 3 mo (29.2)	BL STI: 18.1%	% new STI (gonorrhea, chlamydia, HIV), laboratory (since previous assessment)	3 6 12	NR NR NR	NR NR NR	NSD NSD NSD
Jemmott (high IG), 2007[79,160] Good	Newark, NJ, primary care	Increased	323	African American women ages 18 to 45 y (27.2)	BL STI: 20.3%	% STI (gonorrhea, chlamydia, trichomoniasis), laboratory	6 12	IG1: 0.18 IG2: 0.16 IG1: 0.15 IG2: 0.19	0.15 0.27	IG1/IG3 vs. CG: p=0.35 IG1/IG3 vs. IG2/IG4: p=0.38 IG1/IG3 vs. CG: p=0.03 IG1/IG3 vs. IG2/IG4: p=0.13
Carey, 2004[64] Fair	Syracuse, NY, psychiatric clinic	Increased	408	Adults age ≥18 y with a mood or thought disorder and alcohol or drug use in past year (36.5)	Lifetime: 38%	% STI (NR), self-reported	BL 6	10 2	CG1: 8 CG2: 7 CG1: 8 CG2: 5	NR CG1: p<0.013 CG2: p<0.046
Kamb (high IG) 1998[58,144-147] Fair	5 US cities, STI clinic	Increased	2369 (subgroup)	Adults age ≥20 y or older (NR)	BL STI: 32%*	% STI (chlamydia, gonorrhea, syphilis, HIV), laboratory	12	IG1: 10.2	12.0	Ages 20–25 y: IG1 vs. CG: 0.82 (0.53 to 1.2) Age >25 y: IG1 vs. CG: 0.79 (0.54 to 1.16)
Marion, 2009[85] Fair	Chicago, IL, primary care	Prior STI	342	Low-income African American women age ≥18 y with ≥2 STIs in the past year (38.1)	BL STI: 75%	% STI (gonorrhea, chlamydia, trichomoniasis, HIV), laboratory	3	63	67.5	NR
Shain, 2004[73,167] Fair	San Antonio, TX, STI clinic	Prior STI	775	Mexican American and African American women ages 15 to 45 y with 1 of 4 STIs (21.0)	BL STI: 100%	% STI (gonorrhea, chlamydia), laboratory	12 24	IG1: 25.1 IG2: 20.3 IG1: 37.3 IG2: 34.5	26.8 39.8	IG1 vs. CG: adjusted OR, 0.51 (0.31 to 0.83) IG2 vs. CG: adjusted OR, 0.50 (0.31 to 0.8) IG1 vs. CG: adjusted OR, 0.54 (0.34 to 0.85) IG2 vs. CG: adjusted OR, 0.47 (0.30 to 0.73)
Shain, 1999[57,154-156] Fair	San Antonio, TX, research clinic	Prior STI	313 (subgroup)	Mexican American and African American women ages 19 to 45 with a nonviral STI (NR)	BL STI: 100%	% STI (chlamydia, gonorrhea), laboratory	6 12	8.2 11.7	12.0 17.6	Adjusted OR, 1.53 (0.72 to 3.21) Adjusted OR, 1.61 (0.85 to 3.05)

Appendix C Table 4. Results From Included Studies Targeting Adults—STIs

Author, year Quality	Setting	Risk	N rand	Population (mean age, y)	STI History	Outcome, ascertainment	F/U (mo)	IG Results	CG Results	Between Group Difference: Point Estimate (95% CI) or P-value
Boyer, 1997[88] Fair	San Francisco, CA, STI clinic	Prior STI	393	Heterosexual adults ages 18 to 35 y with previous STI, STI symptoms, or known exposure to STI (NR)	Lifetime STI: 61.8%	% new STI (chlamydia, gonorrhea, syphilis, trichomoniasis, HIV, HSV, HPV, BV), laboratory	6	7.1	4.7	NSD

*Data for entire study , which included adults and adolescents

Abbreviations: BL = baseline; BV = bacterial vaginosis; CG = control group; CI = confidence interval; F/U = followup; HIV = human immunodeficiency virus; HR = hazard ratio; HRR = hazard rate ratio; IG = intervention group; NR = not reported; NSD = no significant difference; OR = odds ratio; rand = randomized; STI = sexually transmitted infection.

Appendix C Table 5. Results From Included Studies Targeting Adolescents—Condom Use and Unprotected Sexual Intercourse

Author, year / Quality	Setting	Risk	N rand	Population (mean age, y)	STI History	Outcome	F/U (mo)	IG Results	CG Results	Between Group Difference: Point Estimate (95% CI) or P-value
Low-intensity (<30 min)										
Boekeloo, 1999[63,143]	Washington DC, primary care	Low/mix	219	Adolescents ages 12 to 15 y (NR)	Treated for STI: 5.9%	% used condom at most recent vaginal intercourse among sexually active	BL	75	69	OR, 1.17 (0.29 to 2.83)
							3	92	57	OR, 18.0 (1.27 to 256.03)
							9	71	70	OR, 1.0 (0.31 to 3.24)
Fair						% unprotected intercourse among sexually active	3	8	43	Adjusted OR, 1.55 (NR†)
Moderate-intensity (30 to 120 minutes)										
Danielson 1990[66]	Portland, OR, and Vancouver, WA, HMO	Low/mix	1195	Adolescent boys ages 15 to 18 y (NR)	NR	% used no contraception at most recent intercourse among sexually active	BL	39.1	39.6	NR
							12	30.1	34.2	NR
Fair						% used condom at most recent intercourse among sexually active	BL	39	36.7	NR
							12	33.6	35.8	p=0.60 (calculated)
High-intensity (>120 minutes)										
Jemmott, 2005[67]	Philadelphia, PA, primary care	Increased	682	Sexually active African American or Latino adolescent girls ages 12 to 19 y (15.5)	BL STI: 21.6%	Number of days of unprotected vaginal intercourse in past 3 mo, mean (SE)	BL	IG1: 3.2 (0.5) IG2: 2.5 (0.5)	3.0 (0.5)	NSD
							3	IG1: 3.6 (0.8) IG2: 3.7 (0.8)	3.5 (0.8)	IG1 vs. CG: p=0.89 / IG2 vs. CG: p=0.95
Good							6	IG1: 2.6 (0.7) IG2: 3.0 (0.7)	3.3 (0.7)	IG1 vs. CG: p=0.43 / IG2 vs. CG: p=0.66
							12	IG1: 4.0 (0.8) IG2: 2.3 (0.8)	5.1 (0.8)	IG1 vs. CG: p=0.32 / IG2 vs. CG: p=0.002
DiClemente, 2004[68,148-153]	Birmingham, AL, primary care	Increased	522	Sexually active African American adolescent girls ages 14 to 18 y (16)	BL STI: G: 5.2% C: 17.4% T: 12.6%	% used condom at most recent intercourse	BL	31.9	32.1	NR
							6	80.7	54.1	OR, 5.08 (2.83 to 9.14)
Good							12	72.3	53.9	OR, 3.32 (1.86 to 5.92) / Adjusted OR, 3.94 (2.58 to 6.03)
						% consistent condom use in past 6 mo	BL	43.5	48.6	NR
							6	61.3	42.6	OR, 2.48 (1.44 to 4.26)
							12	58.1	45.3	OR, 2.14 (1.2 to 3.84) / Adjusted OR, 2.30 (1.51 to 3.50)
						Number of unprotected vaginal intercourse episodes in past 6 mo, mean (SD)	BL	4.81 (16.0)	4.23 (10.3)	NR
							6	3.77 (11.7)	9.24 (23.1)	Adjusted mean difference, -6.51 (-10.97 to -2.9)
							12	5.77 (16.4)	10.25 (24.7)	Adjusted mean difference, -5.51 (-11.18 to -0.34)
Shain, 1999[57,154-156]	San Antonio, TX, research clinic	Prior STI	148 (sub-group)	Mexican American and African American adolescent girls ages 14 to 18 y with a nonviral STI (NR)	BL STI: 100%	% unsafe sex	BL	39.4	43.9	p=0.58
							6	16.7	29.3	p=0.09
Fair							12	36.4	43.9	p=0.40

*Data for entire study population, which included adults and adolescents.
†Reported confidence intervals appear to be erroneous.

Abbreviations: BL = baseline; C = chlamydia; CG = control group; CI = confidence interval; F/U = followup; G = gonorrhea; HIV = human immunodeficiency virus; IG = intervention group; NR = not reported; NSD = no significant difference; OR = odds ratio; rand = randomized; STI = sexually transmitted infection; T = trichomonas.

Appendix C Table 6. Results From Included Studies Targeting Adults—Condom Use and Unprotected Sexual Intercourse

Author, year Quality	Setting	Risk	N rand	Population (mean age, y)	STI History	Outcome	F/U (m)	IG Results	CG Results	Between Group Difference: Point Estimate (95% CI) or P-value
Low-intensity (<30 minutes)										
Proude, 2004[76] Fair	Australia, primary care	General	312	Adults ages 18 to 25 y (NR)	NR	% used condom in first sex with new partner	3	73	77	p=0.813
Scholes, 2003[83] Fair	WA and NC, primary care	General	1210	Sexually active nonmonogamous women ages 18 to 24 y (21)	Lifetime STI: 27%	% consistent use of condoms in past 3 mo with all partners	6	36.8	33.5	Adjusted OR, 1.24 (0.89 to 1.73)
						% any use of condoms in the past 3 mo with any partner	BL	71	73	NSD
							6	72.8	63.0	Adjusted OR, 1.86 (1.32 to 2.65)
						Average % of time condoms used with any partner	BL	54	55	NSD
							6	52.7	47.9	Adjusted OR, 5.2 (0.4 to 10.4)
Carey (low IG) 2010[84,157,158] Fair	Syracuse, NY, STI clinic	Increased	496	Adults age ≥18 y with high-risk behavior in past 3 mo (29.2)	BL STI: 18.1%	Number of unprotected sex episodes in past 3 mo, mean (SD)	BL	IG1: 16.5 (20.1)	16.4 (21.3)	NSD
							3	IG1: 10.6 (15.4)	10.5 (15.1)	NSD
							6	IG1: 14.2 (19.9)	10.6 (15.2)	NSD
							12	IG1: 14 (19.7)	11.6 (17.9)	NSD
Peipert, 2008[72,159] Fair	Providence, RI, primary care and Planned Parenthood	Increased	542	Women ages 13 to 35 y at high risk for STI or unplanned pregnancy due to age, behavior, history of STI, or pregnancy (median, 22)	Lifetime STI: 47%	% consistent condom use	24	46	46	Adjusted HRR, 1.26 (0.88 to 1.79)
Jemmott (low IG), 2007[79,160] Fair	Newark, NJ, primary care	Increased	322	African American women ages 18 to 45 y (27.2)	BL STI: 20.3%	Condom use during last intercourse in the past 3 mo, adjusted mean proportion (SE)	3	IG3: 0.52 (0.02) IG4: 0.51 (0.02)	0.39 (0.03)	IG1/IG3 vs. CG: p=0.05 IG1/IG3 vs. IG2/IG4: p=0.92
							6	IG3: 0.46 (0.02) IG4: 0.59 (0.02)	0.51 (0.03)	IG1/IG3 vs. CG: p=0.89 IG1/IG3 vs. IG2/IG4: p=0.69
							12	IG3: 0.55 (0.02) IG4: 0.52 (0.02)	0.40 (0.03)	IG1/IG3 vs. CG: p=0.03 IG1/IG3 vs. IG2/IG4: p=0.01
						Unprotected sexual intercourse in past 3 mo, during last sexual intercourse in past 3 mo, adjusted mean frequency (SE)	3	IG3: 3.08 (0.46) IG4: 5.40 (0.42)	8.2 (1.62)	IG1/IG3 vs. CG: p=0.02 IG1/IG3 vs. IG2/IG4: p=0.01
							6	IG3: 3.38 (0.51) IG4: 5.58 (0.34)	6.90 (1.47)	IG1/IG3 vs. CG: p=0.59 IG1/IG3 vs. IG2/IG4: p=0.16
							12	IG3: 3.60 (0.64) IG4: 5.12 (0.24)	8.34 (1.90)	IG1/IG3 vs. CG: p=0.18 IG1/IG3 vs. IG2/IG4: p=0.02
Cortes-Bordoy 2010[86] Fair	Spain, gynecology clinic	Prior STI	211	Women age ≥18 y with vulvoperineal warts (30.2)	Lifetime STI: 100%	% reporting condom use in past 3 mo	BL	66.1	77.2	p=0.115
							3	83.2	75.8	p=0.250
							6	76.1	68.7	p=0.301
							9	67.5	65.1	p=0.899
							12	65.4	69.3	p=0.752
Moderate-intensity (30 to 120 min)										
Petersen, 2007[70] Fair	Chapel Hill, NC, primary care	General	764	Women ages 16 to 44 y at risk for unintended pregnancy (no IUD or sterilization) (NR)	NR	Proportion reporting consistent condom use (among those who use condoms) over past 12 mo	12	NR	NR	NSD

Appendix C Table 6. Results From Included Studies Targeting Adults—Condom Use and Unprotected Sexual Intercourse

Author, year Quality	Setting	N rand	Risk	Population (mean age, y)	STI History	Outcome	F/U (m)	IG Results	CG Results	Between Group Difference: Point Estimate (95% CI) or P-value
Wenger, 1992[7] Fair	Los Angeles, CA, primary care	435	General	University students age ≥18 y (23)	Lifetime STI: 23%	% with unprotected intercourse with last sex partner	BL	IG1: 72 / IG2: 70	63	NSD
							6	IG1: 69 / IG2: 63	61	NSD
Metsch, 2013[90] Good	7 states and Washington, DC, STI clinic	5012	Increased	Adults age ≥18 y seeking services at an STI clinic (NR)	BL STI: 44.3%	Number of unprotected sex acts, predicted mean (95% CI)	BL	23.9 (22.1 to 25.9)	22.6 (20.9 to 24.4)	NSD
							6	17.4 (15.5 to 19.4)	18.3 (16.4 to 20.5)	Adjusted risk ratio, 0.98 (0.86 to 1.13)
Berenson (mod IG), 2012[71] Fair	Southeast TX, reproductive health clinic	771	Increased	Sexually active women ages 16 to 24 y (19.9)	Lifetime STI: 26.1%	% condom use at last intercourse	BL	IG1: 47	48.2	p=0.56 (3-way)
							3	IG1: 19.6	21.1	p=0.08 (3-way)
							6	IG1: 12	13.1	p=0.45 (3-way) IG1 vs. CG: OR, 1.12 (0.87 to 1.45)
Kershaw, 2009[59] Fair	Atlanta, GA, and New Haven, CT, primary care	1047	Increased	Pregnant women age <25 y (20.4)	Lifetime STI: "more than half"	Number of acts of unprotected intercourse, mean (SE)	BL	5.26 (6.8)	CG1: 6.45 (8.3) / CG2: 5.66 (7.6)	NR
							3rd tri	4.47 (6.9)	CG1: 5.05 (7.2) / CG2: 4.14 (6.6)	F-test: 0.49; p=0.49
							6	3.81 (6.5)	CG1: 4.84 (7.2) / CG2: 4.72 (7.0)	F-test: 1.79; p=0.18
							12	3.89 (6.5)	CG1: 5.69 (7.9) / CG2: 5.26 (7.8)	F-test: 3.78; p=0.04
						% condom use, mean (SD)	BL	39.29 (37.7)	CG1: 35.54 (37.0) / CG2: 35.93 (38.1)	NR
							3rd tri	34.67 (39.2)	CG1: 31.35 (37.9) / CG2: 29.01 (39.3)	F-test: 1.06; p=0.3
							6	51.03 (40.6)	CG1: 42.74 (39.5) / CG2: 40.67 (40.1)	F-test: 7.45; p=0.007
							12	49.76 (41.4)	CG1: 41.88 (41.3) / CG2: 44.11 (40.8)	F-test: 3.93; p=0.04
Kamb (mod IG), 1998[58,144-147] Fair	5 US cities, STI clinic	2890	Increased	Adults and adolescents age ≥14 y (median, 25)	BL STI: 32%	% no unprotected intercourse in past 3 mo	BL	IG2: 13	13	NR
							3	IG2: 44	38	IG2 vs. CG: adjusted RR, 1.15 (1.03 to 1.27)
							6	IG2: 39	34	IG2 vs. CG: adjusted RR, 1.12 (1.00 to 1.25)
							9	IG2: 43	42	NR
							12	IG2: 41	41	NR
						% reporting any condom use in past 3 mo	BL	IG2: 61	62	NR
							3	IG2: 79	76	NR
							6	IG2: 73	73	NR
Crosby, 2009[87] Fair	Southern US, STI clinic	266	Prior STI	African American men ages 18 to 29 y with newly diagnosed STI and recent experience with condoms (23.2)	BL STI: 100%	% used condom at last intercourse	BL	52.5	42.4	NSD
							3	72.4	53.9	Adjusted OR, 2.2 (1.08 to 4.48)
						Number of unprotected intercourse episodes in past 3 mo, mean (SD)	BL	16.0 (47.3)	14.3 (21.0)	NSD
							3	12.3 (25.8)	29.4 (79.3)	OR, -13.4 (-35.6 to 8.8)
High-intensity (>120 min)										
Berenson (high IG), 2012[71] Fair	Southeast TX, reproductive health clinic	772	Increased	Sexually active women ages 16 to 24 y (19.9)	Lifetime STI: 26.1%	% condom use at last intercourse	BL	IG2: 50.8	48.2	p=0.56 (3-way)
							3	IG2: 26	21.1	p=0.08 (3-way)
							6	IG2: 15.1	13.1	p=0.45 (3-way) IG2 vs. CG: OR, 1.32 (1.03 to 1.70)

Appendix C Table 6. Results From Included Studies Targeting Adults—Condom Use and Unprotected Sexual Intercourse

Author, year Quality	Setting	Risk	N rand	Population (mean age, y)	STI History	Outcome	F/U (m)	IG Results	CG Results	Between Group Difference: Point Estimate (95% CI) or P-value
Cianelli, 2012[75] Fair	Chile, primary care	Increased	496	Chilean women ages 18 to 49 y (32.5)	NR	% any condom use in past 3 mo	BL	22.22	18.32	NR
							3	28.66	21.78	NSD
Carey (high IG), 2010[34,157,158]	Syracuse, NY, STI clinic	Increased	1235	Adults age ≥18 y with high-risk behavior in past 3 mo (29.2)	BL STI: 18.1%	Number of unprotected sex episodes in past 3 mo, mean (SD)	BL	IG2: 15.3 (19.2) IG3: 16.7 (21.1) IG4: 20.4 (24.2) IG5: 18.6 (21.3)	16.4 (21.3)	NSD
Fair							3	IG2: 12.1 (16.6) IG3: 12.3 (17.0) IG4: 12 (16.6) IG5: 12.5 (17.2)	10.5 (15.1)	NSD
							6	IG2: 11.3 (16.3) IG3: 14.4 (19.2) IG4: 15.1 (20.3) IG5: 14.1 (19.8)	10.6 (15.2)	NSD
							12	IG2: 13.1 (17.8) IG3: 15.7 (22.1) IG4: 13.9 (19.6) IG5: 15 (20.8)	11.6 (17.9)	NSD
Berkman, 2007[82] Good	NY, psychiatric clinic	Increased	149	Adult males ages 18 to 59 y with severe mental illness (38.6)	NR	% of time condoms used during sex among sexually active at BL in past 3 mo	BL	81.6	70.7	t-test: 0.98; p=0.33
							6	93.4	75.8	t-test: 1.95; p=0.06
							12	82.9	76.5	t-test: 0.57; p=0.57
Jemmott (high IG), 2007[79,160]	Newark, NJ, primary care	Increased	323	African American women ages 18 to 45 y (27.2)	BL STI: 20.3%	Condom use during last intercourse in the past 3 mo, adjusted mean proportion (SE)	3	IG1: 0.52 (0.02) IG2: 0.51 (0.02)	0.39 (0.03)	IG1/IG3 vs. CG: p=0.05 / IG1/IG3 vs. IG2/IG4: p=0.92
Fair							6	IG1: 0.6 (0.02) IG2: 0.46 (0.02)	0.51 (0.03)	IG1/IG3 vs. CG: p=0.89 / IG1/IG3 vs. IG2/IG4: p=0.69
							12	IG1: 0.59 (0.02) IG2: 0.36 (0.02)	0.40 (0.03)	IG1/IG3 vs. CG: p=0.03 / IG1/IG3 vs. IG2/IG4: p=0.01
						Unprotected sexual intercourse in the past 3 mo, during last sexual intercourse in past 3 mo, adjusted mean frequency (SE)	3	IG1: 4.49 (0.73) IG2: 5.32 (0.54)	8.2 (1.62)	IG1/IG3 vs. CG: p=0.02 / IG1/IG3 vs. IG2/IG4: p=0.01
							6	IG1: 4.93 (0.73) IG2: 3.77 (0.34)	6.90 (1.47)	IG1/IG3 vs. CG: p=0.59 / IG1/IG3 vs. IG2/IG4: p=0.16
							12	IG1: 5.14 (0.89) IG2: 5.94 (0.62)	8.34 (1.90)	IG1/IG3 vs. CG: p=0.18 / IG1/IG3 vs. IG2/IG4: p=0.02
Carey, 2004[64] Fair	Syracuse, NY, psychiatric clinic	Increased	408	Adults age ≥18 y with a mood or thought disorder and alcohol or drug use in past year (36.5)	Lifetime STI: 38%	Number of unprotected intercourse acts in past 3 mo, mean (SD)	BL	14 (31.2)	CG: 10.8 (22.1) CG2: 11.6 (25.9)	NSD
							5w	8.7 (14.5)	CG1: 9.4 (22.9) CG2: 12.1 (25.6)	NR
							3	9.5 (23.1)	CG1: 8.1 (20.3) CG2: 10 (21.1)	NR
							6	7.2 (14.5)	CG1: 8.8 (20.2) CG2: 8.0 (17.9)	Condition x time interaction, IG vs. CG1: p=0.001 Condition x time interaction, IG vs. CG2: p=0.004
Ehrhardt, 2002[81,105,163-166] Good	Brooklyn, NY, Planned Parenthood	Increased	360	Women ages 18 to 30 y (22.26)	Past 3-mo STI: 16.9%	Number of unprotected intercourse occasions	1	NR	NR	IG1 vs. CG: 3.5; p=0.09 IG2 vs. CG: 2; p=0.2
							12	NR	NR	IG1 vs. CG: 4; p=0.00 IG2 vs. CG: NR; NSD

Appendix C Table 6. Results From Included Studies Targeting Adults—Condom Use and Unprotected Sexual Intercourse

Author, year Quality	Setting	Risk	N rand	Population (mean age, y)	STI History	Outcome	F/U (m)	IG Results	CG Results	Between Group Difference: Point Estimate (95% CI) or P-value
Kamb (high IG), 1998[58,144,147]	5 US cities, STI clinic	Increased	2881	Adults and adolescents age ≥14 y (25 median)	BL STI: 32%	% no unprotected intercourse in past 3 mo	BL	IG1: 16	13	NR
							3	IG1: 46	38	IG1 vs. CG: adjusted RR, 1.21 (1.09 to 1.35)
Fair							6	IG1: 39	34	IG1 vs. CG: adjusted RR, 1.14 (1.01 to 1.28)
							9	IG1: 44	42	NR
							12	IG1: 42	41	NR
					% reporting any condom use in past 3 mo	BL	IG1: 63	62	NR
						3	IG1: 83 (IG2: 79)	76	IG1 vs. CG: p<0.05 / IG1 vs. IG2: p<0.05
						6	IG1: 78 (IG2: 73)	73	IG1 vs. CG: p<0.05 / IG1 vs. IG2: p<0.05
Shain, 2004[73,167]	San Antonio, TX, STI clinic	Prior STI	775	Mexican American and African American women ages 15 to 45 y with 1 of 4 STIs (21.0)	BL STI: 100%	% unprotected sex with untreated or incompletely treated partner	12	IG1: 7.8 IG2: 10.2	18.1	IG1 vs. CG: p=0.001 / IG2 vs. CG: p=0.01
Fair										
Shain, 1999[57,154-156]	San Antonio, TX, research clinic	Prior STI	313 (sub-group)	Mexican American and African American women ages 19 to 45 y with a nonviral STI (21.6)	BL STI: 100%	% unsafe sex	BL	42.7	35.2	p=0.18
Fair							6	19.9	28.2	p=0.04
							12	25.7	42.3	p<0.001
Boyer, 1997[88]	San Francisco, CA, STI clinic	Prior STI	393	Heterosexual adults ages 18 to 35 y with previous STI, STI symptoms, or known exposure to STI (NR)	Lifetime STI: 61.8%	% no sexual encounters without condom	BL	11.7	15.7	NR
Fair							3	40.5	31.1	NR
							5	39.1	30.7	NR

Abbreviations: BL = baseline; BV = bacterial vaginosis; C = chlamydia; CG = control group; CI = confidence interval; F/U = followup; G = gonorrhea; HIV = human immunodeficiency virus; HR = hazard ratio; HRR = hazard rate ratio; IG = intervention group; NR = not reported; NSD = no significant difference; OR = odds ratio; rand = randomized; STI = sexually transmitted infection; T = trichomoniasis.

Appendix C Table 7. Results From Included Studies Targeting Adolescents—Other Sexual Behavioral Outcomes

Author, year Quality	Setting	Risk	N rand	Population	STI History	Outcome	F/U (mo)	IG Results	CG Results	Between Group Difference: Point Estimate (95% CI) or P-value
Low-intensity (<30 min)										
Boekeloo, 1999[63,143] Fair	Washington DC, primary care	Low/mix	219	Adolescents ages 12 to 15 y	Treated for STI: 5.9%	% vaginal intercourse in past 3 mo	BL	20	23	OR, 0.90 (0.28 to 2.83)
							3	27	20	OR, 2.46 (1.04 to 5.84)
							9	33	29	OR, 1.64 (0.81 to 3.34)
Moderate-intensity (30 to 120 min)										
Guilamo-Ramos, 2011[65] Fair	New York, NY, primary care	Low/mix	264	African American and Latino adolescents ages 11 to 14 y	NR	% any vaginal intercourse	BL	6.9	6.4	NR
							9	6.8	22.2	p<0.05
High-intensity (>120 min)										
Jemmott, 2005[67] Fair	Philadelphia, PA, primary care	Increased	682	Sexually active African American or Latino adolescent girls ages 12 to 19 y	BL STI: 21.6%	Number of sexual partners in past 3 mo, adjusted mean (SE)	BL	IG1: 1.14 (0.05) IG2: 1.04 (0.05)	1.11 (0.04)	NR
							3	IG1: 1.04 (0.06) IG2: 0.97 (0.06)	1.07 (0.07)	IG1 vs. CG: p=0.490 IG2 vs. CG: p=0.13 IG1 vs. IG2: p=0.41
							6	IG1: 0.98 (0.06) IG2: 0.92 (0.06)	1.00 (0.06)	IG1 vs. CG: p=0.56 IG2 vs. CG: p=0.22 IG1 vs. IG2: p=0.53
							12	IG1: 1.00 (0.05) IG2: 0.91 (0.05)	1.04 (0.05)	IG1 vs. CG: p=0.51 IG2 vs. CG: p=0.04 IG1 vs. IG2: p=0.17
						% ≥2 sex partners in past 3 mo, adjusted mean (SE)	BL	IG1: 18.9 (NR) IG2: 12.3 (NR)	16.4 (NR)	NR
							3	IG1: 15.1 (2.4) IG2: 10.9 (2.4)	14.2 (2.5)	IG1 vs. CG: p=0.76 IG2 vs. CG: p=0.29 IG1 vs. IG2: p=0.17
							6	IG1: 12.5 (2.5) IG2: 9.7 (2.5)	14.3 (2.4)	IG1 vs. CG: p=0.54 IG2 vs. CG: p=0.12 IG1 vs. IG2: p=0.36
							12	IG1: 10.7 (2.5) IG2: 6.9 (2.5)	16.6 (2.5)	IG1 vs. CG: p=0.09 IG2 vs. CG: p=0.002 IG1 vs. IG2: p=0.20
						Number of days of sex while under the influence of drugs or alcohol, adjusted mean (SE)	BL	IG1: 0.55 (0.21) IG2: 0.26 (0.10)	0.61 (0.20)	NR
							3	IG1: 0.29 (0.09) IG2: 0.10 (0.09)	0.26 (0.09)	IG1 vs. CG: p=0.98 IG2 vs. CG: p=0.03 IG1 vs. IG2: p=0.03
							6	IG1: 0.15 (0.10) IG2: 0.07 (0.10)	0.31 (0.10)	IG1 vs. CG: p=0.10 IG2 vs. CG: p=0.005 IG1 vs. IG2: p=0.26
							12	IG1: 0.53 (0.25) IG2: 0.42 (0.25)	0.66 (0.25)	IG1 vs. CG: p=0.65 IG2 vs. CG: p=0.37 IG1 vs. IG2: p=0.65
DiClemente, 2004[68,148-153] Good	Birmingham, AL, primary care	Increased	522	Sexually active African American adolescent girls ages 14 to 18 y	BL STI: G: 5.2% C: 17.4% T: 12.6%	% new vaginal sex partner, past 30 days	BL	4.4	7.4	NR
							6	2.7	7.4	OR, 0.29 (0.11 to 0.77)
							12	3.6	5.6	OR, 0.59 (0.19 to 1.84)
						Frequency of vaginal sex, adjusted number of events	6	14.23	17.08	GEE OR, 0.40 (0.19 to 0.82) Relative change, -16.73 (-45.08 to 24.98)
							12	15.82	18.86	Relative change, -16.14 (-39.57 to 7.29)

Appendix C Table 7. Results From Included Studies Targeting Adolescents—Other Sexual Behavioral Outcomes

Author, year Quality	Setting	Risk	N rand	Population	STI History	Outcome	F/U (mo)	IG Results	CG Results	Between Group Difference: Point Estimate (95% CI) or P-value
Shain, 1999[57,] [154-156]	San Antonio, TX, research clinic	Prior STI	148 (sub-group)	Mexican American and African American adolescent girls ages 14 to 18 y with a nonviral STI	BL STI: 100%	% not mutually monogamous	BL	68.2	69.5	p=0.86
							6	37.9	48.8	p=0.18
							12	57.6	69.5	p=0.12
Fair						% rapid partner turnover	6	12.1	23.2	p=0.08
							12	21.2	35.4	p=0.06

*Data for entire study population, which included adults and adolescents.

Abbreviations: BL = baseline; C = chlamydia; CG = control group; CI = confidence interval; F/U = followup; G = gonorrhea; HIV = human immunodeficiency virus; IG = intervention group; NR = not reported; NSD = no significant difference; OR = odds ratio; rand = randomized; STI = sexually transmitted infection; T = trichomoniasis.

Appendix C Table 8. Results From Included Studies Targeting Adults—Other Sexual Behavioral Outcomes

Author, year Quality	Setting	Risk	N rand	Population	STI History	Outcome	F/U (mo)	IG Results	CG Results	Between Group Difference: Point Estimate (95% CI) or P-value
Low-intensity (<30 min)										
Proude, 2004[76] Fair	Australia, primary care	General	312	Adults ages 18 to 25 y	NR	% new sex partners in past 3 mo	3	7	8	NSD
Carey (low IG), 2010[84,157,158] Fair	Syracuse, NY, STI clinic	Increased	496	Adults age ≥18 y with high-risk behavior in past 3 mo	BL STI: 18.1%	Number of sex partners in past 3 mo, mean (SD)	BL 3 6 12	IG1: 2.9 (2.3) IG1: 2.2 (1.8) IG1: 2.1 (2.0) IG1: 1.9 (1.5)	3.0 (2.8) 2.2 (2.1) 2.1 (1.8) 1.9 (1.5)	NSD NSD NSD NSD
Cortes-Bordoy, 2010[86] Fair	Spain, gynecology clinic	Prior STI	211	Women age ≥18 y with vulvoperineal warts	Lifetime STI: 22.7%	Number of sex partners in past 3 mo, mean	BL 3 6 9 12	1.68 0.90 0.95 0.85 0.87	2.08 1.03 1.08 1.05 1.13	p=0.111 p<0.05 p<0.05 p<0.05 p<0.001
Moderate-intensity (30 to 120 min)										
Wenger, 1992[77] Fair	Los Angeles, CA, primary care	General	435	University students age ≥18 y	Lifetime STI: 23%	Number of sex partners in past mo, mean (SD) % ≥2 sex partners in past mo	BL 6 6	IG1: 0.76 (0.61) IG2: 0.82 (0.76) IG1: 0.70 (0.57) IG2: 0.82 (0.76) (data NR by group)	0.82 (0.66) 0.72 (0.58)	NSD NSD NSD
Metsch, 2013[90] Good	7 states and Washington, DC, STI clinics	Increased	5012	Adults age ≥18 y seeking services at an STI clinic (NR)	BL STI: 43.3%	Number of partners, predicted mean (95% CI) Number of unprotected partners, predicted mean (95% CI)	BL 6 BL 6	IG1: 4.7 (4.4 to 4.9) IG1: 2.7 (2.5 to 2.8) 2.1 (2.0 to 2.3) 1.1 (1.0 to 1.2)	4.6 (4.4 to 4.9) 3.0 (2.8 to 3.2) 2.1 (2.0 to 2.2) 1.1 (1.1 to 1.2)	NSD Adjusted risk ratio, 0.88 (0.82 to 0.94) NSD Adjusted risk ratio, 0.97 (0.90 to 1.05)
Berenson (mod IG), 2012[71] Fair	Southeast TX, reproductive health clinic	Increased	771	Sexually active women ages 16 to 24 y	Lifetime STI: 26.1%	% dual use oral birth control and condom at last sexual intercourse % no birth control method at last sexual intercourse	3 6 3 6	IG1: 9.4 IG1: 5.7 IG1: 11.0 IG1: 16.7	11.6 7.2 8.5 13.4	NR OR, 1.01 (0.75 to 1.37) NR OR, 1.26 (0.93 to 1.70)
Kamb (mod IG), 1998[58,144-147] Fair	5 US cities, STI clinic	Increased	2890	Adults and adolescents age ≥14 y	BL STI: 32%	% 0–1 casual or new partners	3 6	IG2: 72 IG2: 70	66 66	IG2 vs. CG: p<0.05
Crosby, 2009[87] Fair	Southern US, STI clinic	Prior STI	266	African American men ages 18 to 29 y with newly diagnosed STI and recent experience with condoms	BL STI: 100%	Number of sex partners in past 3 mo, mean (SD)	3	2.06 (1.65)	4.15 (5.59)	OR, -2.09 (-3.18 to -0.99)
High-intensity (>120 min)										
Berenson (high IG), 2012[71] Fair	Southeast TX, reproductive health clinic	Increased	772	Sexually active women ages 16 to 24 y	Lifetime STI: 26.1%	% dual use oral birth control and condom at last sexual intercourse % no birth control method at last sexual intercourse	3 6 3 6	IG2: 12.5 IG2: 8.3 IG2: 6.0 IG2: 12.8	11.6 7.2 8.5 13.4	NR OR, 1.14 (0.85 to 1.53) NR OR, 0.86 (0.62 to 1.19)

Appendix C Table 8. Results From Included Studies Targeting Adults—Other Sexual Behavioral Outcomes

Author, year Quality	Setting	Risk	N rand	Population	STI History	Outcome	F/U (mo)	IG Results	CG Results	Between Group Difference: Point Estimate (95% CI) or P-value
Carey (high IG), 2010[84,157,158] Fair	Syracuse, NY, STI clinic	Increased	1235	Adults age ≥18 y with high-risk behavior in past 3 mo	BL STI: 18.1%	Number of sex partners in past 3 mo, mean (SD)	BL	IG2: 2.8 (2.3) IG3: 2.7 (2.0) IG4: 2.7 (2.1) IG5: 2.8 (2.3)	3.0 (2.8)	NSD
							3	IG2: 2.1 (1.9) IG3: 2.0 (1.8) IG4: 1.9 (1.8) IG5: 2.0 (1.8)	2.2 (2.1)	NSD
							6	IG2: 2.1 (2.0) IG3: 2.0 (1.8) IG4: 1.7 (1.3) IG5: 2.1 (2.2)	2.1 (1.8)	NSD
							12	IG2: 2.0 (1.7) IG3: 2.0 (1.4) IG4: 1.7 (1.3) IG5: 1.9 (1.6)	1.9 (1.5)	NSD
Berkman, 2007[82] Good	NY, psychiatric clinic	Increased	149	Adult males ages 18 to 59 y with severe mental illness	NR	Number of vaginal equivalent episodes with casual partners in past 6 mo, mean (SD)	BL	0.19 (0.72)	0.60 (2.25)	t=1.49; p=0.140
							6	0.16 (0.60)	0.50 (1.80)	t=1.52; p=0.132
							12	0.29 (0.90)	0.57 (2.00)	t=1.11; p=0.27
Carey, 2004[84] Fair	Syracuse, NY, psychiatric clinic	Increased	408	Adults age ≥18 y with a mood or thought disorder and alcohol or drug use in past year	Lifetime STI: 38%	Number of sex partners, mean (SD)	BL	1.25 (1.11)	CG1: 1.41 (1.67) CG2: 1.24 (1.12)	NR
							5w	1.04 (0.84)	CG1: 1.12 (1.12) CG2: 1.19 (1.29)	NR
							3	0.93 (0.80)	CG1: 1.02 (1.12) CG2: 1.12 (1.16)	NR
							6	0.97 (0.78)	CG1: 0.95 (0.99) CG2: 1.07 (0.38)	Condition x time interaction: IG vs. CG1: p=0.339 IG vs. CG2: p=0.037
						Number of casual sex partners, mean (SD)	BL	0.54 (1.05)	CG1: 0.63 (1.31) CG2: 0.49 (1.05)	NR
							5w	0.28 (0.60)	CG1: 0.38 (0.79) CG2: 0.52 (1.21)	NR
							3	0.21 (0.57)	CG1: 0.33 (0.93) CG2: 0.47 (0.97)	NR
							6	0.30 (0.58)	CG1: 0.30 (0.67) CG2: 0.48 (1.19)	Condition x time interaction: IG vs. CG1: p=0.015 IG vs. CG2: p=0.001
Ehrhardt, 2002[81,105,163-166] Good	Brooklyn, NY, Planned Parenthood	Increased	360	Women ages 18 to 30 y	Past 3-mo STI: 16.9%	% maintaining or improving safer sex	1	IG1: 74.5 IG2: 72.4	60.2	IG1 vs. CG: OR, 1.93 (1.07 to 3.48) IG2 vs. CG: OR, 1.74 (0.99 to 3.04); p=0.05
							12	IG1: 72.7 IG2: 66.4	61.7	IG1 vs. CG: OR, 1.65 (0.94 to 2.90) IG2 vs. CG: OR, 1.22 (0.72 to 2.08)
						% using alternative risk reduction strategies, including leaving relationship, refusing sex, mutual HIV testing, others	1	IG1: NR IG2: NR	NR	IG1 vs. CG: OR, 2.57 (1.2 to 5.51) IG2 vs. CG: OR, 1.77 (0.83 to 3.8)
							12	IG1: 18 IG2: NR	NR	NR

Appendix C Table 8. Results From Included Studies Targeting Adults—Other Sexual Behavioral Outcomes

Author, year Quality	Setting	Risk	N rand	Population	STI History	Outcome	F/U (mo)	IG Results	CG Results	Between Group Difference: Point Estimate (95% CI) or P-value
Kamb (high IG), 1998[58,144-147] Fair	5 US cities, STI clinic	Increased	2881	Adults and adolescents age ≥14 y	BL STI: 32%	% 0–1 casual or new partners	3 6	IG1: 71 IG1: 70	66 66	IG1 vs. CG: p<0.05
Marion, 2009[85] Fair	Chicago, IL, primary care	Prior STI	342	Low-income African American women age ≥18 y with ≥2 STIs in the past year	BL STI: 75%	STI risk index, mean (SD)	BL 3	6.81 (2.6) 4.47 (2)	6.59 (2.2) 6.06 (2.1)	NR t=5.19; p<0.001
Shain, 2004[167] Fair	San Antonio, TX, STI clinic	Prior STI	775	Mexican American and African American women ages 15 to 45 y with 1 of 4 STIs	BL STI: 100%	% 0 or 1 sex partners	12	IG1: 57.5 IG2: 56.8	44.7	NR
							24	IG1: 62.4 IG2: 63.8	49.2	NR
						% ≥2 sex partners	12	IG1: 42.5 IG2: 43.2	55.3	IG1 vs. CG: p=0.001 IG2 vs. CG: p=0.01
							24	IG1: 37.6 IG2: 36.2	50.8	IG1 vs. CG: p<0.005 IG2 vs. CG: p<0.002
Shain, 1999[154-156] Fair	San Antonio, TX, research clinic		617	Mexican American and African American women ages 14 to 45 y with nonviral STI	BL STI: 100%	% 0 or 1 sex partners % >1 sex partners	12 12	67.5 32.5	56.1 43.9	NR p=0.004
Boyer, 1997[88] Fair	San Francisco, CA, STI clinic	Prior STI	393	Heterosexual adults ages 18 to 35 y with previous STI, STI symptoms, or known exposure to STI	Lifetime STI: 61.8%	% ≥2 sexual encounters with nonsteady partner	3 and/or 5	18.8	25.2	NR

Abbreviations: BL = baseline; CG = control group; CI = confidence interval; F/U = followup; HIV = human immunodeficiency virus; IG = intervention group; NR = not reported; NSD = no significant difference; OR = odds ratio; rand = randomized; STI = sexually transmitted infection.

Appendix C Table 9. Results From Included Studies Targeting Adolescents—Other Positive Outcomes

Author, year Quality	Setting	Risk	N rand	Population	STI History	Outcome	F/U (mo)	IG Results	CG Results	Between Group Difference: Point Estimate (95% CI) or P-value
Low-intensity (<30 min)										
Boekeloo, 1999[83,143] Fair	Washington DC, primary care	Low/mix	219	Adolescents ages 12 to 15 y	Treated for STI: 5.9%	% gotten someone or been pregnant	BL	1	1.8	NSD
							3	0	1.9	NSD
							9	1.1	5.9	NSD
Moderate-intensity (30 to 120 min)										
Danielson, 1990[66] Fair	Portland, OR and Vancouver, WA, HMO	Low/mix	1195	Adolescent boys ages 15 to 18 y	NR	% performing testicular self-exam ≥3 times in past year	12	30	11	NR
						% used an effective form of birth control at last intercourse	12	65.8	64.6	OR, 1.51; p<0.05
High-intensity (>120 min)										
DiClemente, 2004[68, 148-153] Good	Birmingham, AL, primary care	Increased	522	Sexually active African American adolescent girls ages 14 to 18 y	BL STI: G: 5.2% C: 17.4% T: 12.6%	% pregnant	6	3.6	7.0	OR, 0.38 (0.15 to 0.36)
							12	6.0	8.5	OR, 0.74 (0.3 to 1.82) GEE OR, 0.53 (0.27 to 1.03)

Abbreviations: BL = baseline; C = chlamydia; CG = control group; CI = confidence interval; F/U = followup; G = gonorrhea; HIV = human immunodeficiency virus; IG = intervention group; NR = not reported; NSD = no significant difference; OR = odds ratio; rand = randomized; STI = sexually transmitted infection; T = trichomoniasis.

Appendix C Table 10. Results From Included Studies Targeting Adults—Other Positive Outcomes

Author, year Quality	Setting	Risk	N rand	Population	STI History	Outcome	F/U (mo)	IG Results	CG Results	Between Group Difference: Point Estimate (95% CI) or P-value
Low-intensity (<30 min)										
Peipert, 2008[72,159] Fair	Providence, RI, primary care and Planned Parenthood	Increased	542	Women ages 13 to 35 y at high risk for STI or unplanned pregnancy due to age, behavior, history of STI or pregnancy	Lifetime STI: 47%	% unplanned pregnancy	24	22	23	Adjusted HRR for dual method and propensity score: 1.22 (0.73 to 2.04)
Moderate-intensity (30 to 120 min)										
Petersen, 2007[70] Fair	Chapel Hill, NC, primary care	General	764	Women ages 16 to 44 y at risk for unintended pregnancy (no IUD or sterilization)	NR	% unintended pregnancy	12	10 (data NR by group)	(data NR by group)	NSD
						% improved or maintained an ongoing level of contraceptive use	BL	59	58	NSD
							2	72	66	NSD
							8	63	62	NSD
							12	64	60	NSD
Berenson (mod IG), 2012[71] Fair	Southeast TX, reproductive health clinic	Increased	771	Sexually active women ages 16 to 24 y	Lifetime STI: 26.1%	% pregnant	12	IG1: 16.4	12.4	IG1 vs. CG: HR, 1.39 (0.95 to 2.03)
Kershaw, 2009[59] Fair	Atlanta, GA, and New Haven, CT, primary care	Increased	1047	Pregnant women age <25 y	Lifetime STI: "more than half"	% repeat pregnancy	6	5.6	CG1: 7.9 CG2: 12.9	OR, 0.49 (0.27 to 0.91)
							12	23.1	CG1: 22.5 CG2: 26.0	OR, 0.95 (0.63 to 1.78)
High-intensity (>120 min)										
Berenson (high IG), 2012[71] Fair	Southeast TX, reproductive health clinic	Increased	772	Sexually active women ages 16 to 24 y	Lifetime STI: 26.1%	% pregnant	12	IG2: 13.5	12.4	IG2 vs. CG: HR, 1.07 (0.72 to 1.59)
Cianelli, 2012[75] Fair	Chile, primary care	Increased	496	Chilean women ages 18 to 49 y	NR	CES-D depressive symptoms, mean (SD)	BL	23.27 (11.8)	21.82 (11.1)	NR
							3	21.91 (10.4)	22.28 (11.8)	Multiple regression coefficient: t = -2.24; p<0.05
Ehrhardt, 2002[81,105,163-166] Good	Brooklyn, NY, Planned Parenthood	Increased	360	Women ages 18 to 30 y	Past 3-mo STI: 16.9%	% women reporting physical abuse	1	IG1: 7 IG2: 16	11	NSD
							6	IG1: 18 IG2: 12	18	NSD
							12	IG1: 13 IG2: 9	11	NSD

Abbreviations: BL = baseline; CG = control group; CI = confidence interval; F/U = followup; IG = intervention group; NR = not reported; NSD = no significant difference; OR = odds ratio; rand = randomized; STI = sexually transmitted infection.

Appendix C Table 11. Selected Methodological Quality Indicators From Included Studies Targeting Adolescents (Excluding Subgroup Analyses)

Intervention Intensity	Author, year	Risk	N rand	Quality Rating	Valid Random Assignment	Allocation Concealment	Blind Outcomes Assessment	Objective Biological Outcome	Study Retention, 12 mo or Closest (%)
Low (<30 min)	Boekeloo, 1999[63,143]	Low/mix	219	Fair	(--)	(--)	Yes	No	IG: 90 CG: 90
Moderate (30 to120 min)	Guilamo-Ramos, 2011[65]	Low/mix	264	Fair	(--)	(--)	(Self-admin)	No	IG: 93 CG: 96
	Danielson, 1990[66]	Low/mix	1195	Fair	No	(--)	Yes	No	IG: 83 CG: 82
High (>120 min)	Jemmott, 2005[67]	Increased	682	Fair	Yes	(--)	Yes	Yes	IG1: 86 IG2: 89 CG: 91
	DiClemente, 2004[68,148-153]	Increased	522	Good	Yes	Yes	Yes	Yes	IG: 87 CG: 89
	Champion, 2012[69]	Prior STI	559	Fair	Yes	Yes	(--)	Yes	IG: 73 CG: 73

Abbreviations: CG = control group; IG = intervention group; rand = randomized; STI = sexually transmitted infection.

Appendix C Table 12. Selected Methodological Quality Indicators From Included Studies Targeting Adults (Excluding Subgroup Analyses)

Intervention Intensity	Author, year Quality	Risk	N rand	Quality Rating	Valid Random Assignment	Allocation Concealment	Blind Outcomes Assessment	Objective Biological Outcome	Study Retention, 12m or Closest (%)
Low (<30 min)	Proude, 2004[76]	General	312	Fair	(--)	Yes	(Mailed)	No	IG: 66 CG: 69
	Scholes, 2003[83]	General	1210	Fair	(--)	(--)	No	No	IG: 88 CG: 85
	Carey (low IG), 2010[84,157,158]	Increased	1483	Fair	Yes	(--)	(Computer-admin)	Yes	IG1: 73 CG: 69
	Peipert, 2008[72,159]	Increased	542	Fair	Yes	Yes	Yes	Yes	IG: 61 CG: 67
	Warner, 2006[78]	Increased	40,282	Good	Yes	(--)	(--)	Yes	IG: 96 CG: 96
	Jemmott (low IG), 2007[79,160]	Increased	564	Good	Yes	Yes	Yes	Yes	IG3: 85 IG4: 86 CG: 83
	Marrazzo, 2011[74,161,162]	Prior STI	89	Fair	Yes	Yes	(--)	Yes	IG: 94 CG: 88
	Cortes-Bordoy, 2010[86]	Prior STI	211	Fair	(--)	(--)	No	Yes	(--)
Moderate (30 to120 min)	Petersen, 2007[70]	General	764	Fair	Yes	Yes	(--)	Yes	87 overall
	Wenger, 1992[77]	General	435	Fair	(--)	Yes	(Mailed)	No	IG1: 91 IG2: 90 CG: 81
	Metsch, 2013[90]	Increased	5012	Good	Yes	(--)	(--)	Yes	IG: 86.9 CG: 86.9
	Berenson (mod IG), 2012[71]	Increased	1155	Fair	Yes	Yes	Yes	Partial	IG1: 70 CG: 69
	Neumann, 2011[80]	Increased	3365	Fair	(--)	(--)	(Self-admin)	Yes	(--)
	Kershaw, 2009[59]	Increased	1047	Fair	Yes	(--)	(Computer-admin)	Yes	IG: 82 CG1: 81 CG2: 78
	Kamb (mod IG), 1998[58,144-147]	Increased	5758	Fair	Yes	Yes	Yes	Yes	66 overall
	Crosby, 2009[87]	Prior STI	266	Fair	Yes	Yes	(Self-admin)	Yes	IG: 74 CG: 74
High (>120 min)	Wingood, 2013[89]	Increased	848	Good	Yes	Yes	Yes	Yes	IG: 87 CG: 91
	Berenson (high IG), 2012[71]	Increased	1155	Fair	Yes	Yes	Yes	Partial	IG2: 72 CG: 69
	Cianelli, 2012[75]	Increased	496	Fair	(--)	(--)	(--)	No	IG: 75 CG:86
	Carey (high IG), 2010[84,157,158]	Increased	1483	Fair	Yes	(--)	(Computer-admin)	Yes	IG2: 70 IG3: 68 IG4: 70 IG5: 71 CG: 69
	Berkman, 2007[82]	Increased	149	Good	Yes	Yes	Yes	No	85 overall
	Jemmott (high IG), 2007[79,160]	Increased	564	Good	Yes	Yes	Yes	Yes	IG1: 86 IG2: 94 CG: 83

Appendix C Table 12. Selected Methodological Quality Indicators From Included Studies Targeting Adults (Excluding Subgroup Analyses)

Intervention Intensity	Author, year Quality	Risk	N rand	Quality Rating	Valid Random Assignment	Allocation Concealment	Blind Outcomes Assessment	Objective Biological Outcome	Study Retention, 12m or Closest (%)
	Carey, 2004[64]	Increased	408	Fair	(--)	(--)	Yes	No	IG: 87 CG1: 86 CG2: 87
	Ehrhardt, 2002[81,105,163-166]	Increased	360	Good	Yes	Yes	Yes	No	IG1: 98 IG2: 96 CG: 96
	Kamb (high IG), 1998[58,144-147]	Increased	5758	Fair	Yes	Yes	Yes	Yes	66 overall
	Marion, 2009[85]	Prior STI	342	Fair	Yes	Yes	Yes	Yes	IG: 63 CG: 76
	Shain, 2004[73,167]	Prior STI	775	Fair	(NR)	Yes	No	Yes	IG1: 90 IG2: 91 CG: 93
	Shain, 1999[57,154-156]	Prior STI	617	Fair	(NR)	Yes	No	Yes	IG: 91 CG: 87
	Boyer, 1997[88]	Prior STI	393	Fair	Yes	Yes	No	Yes	60 overall

Abbreviations: CG = control group; IG = intervention group; rand = randomized; STI = sexually transmitted infection.

Appendix D. Ongoing or Recently Completed Studies

Study Country	Aim	Population (n)	Intervention Description	Control Description	Relevant Outcomes	Status
Arnold, 2012[168] (Bruthas Project) United States	To evaluate the effect of the Bruthas Project and determine efficacy of the intervention at reducing HIV risk behavior among black men who have sex with men and women	Adult black men who have sex with men (400)	Semistructured, individualized risk reduction counseling sessions, HIV counseling and testing	Standard HIV counseling and testing	Sexual risk behavior	Estimated completion, December 2014
Brady, 2010[169] United States	To determine whether a motivational interviewing and skills building intervention reduces HIV risk behavior in adults with mental illness	Adults with a mental illness (60)	Motivational interviewing to decrease HIV risk behaviors in addition to information and skill building	HIV information and skill building	Unprotected sexual activity, sex while under the influence	Completed, October 2008
Brady, 2012[170] United States	To examine the effectiveness of a brief, tailored primary and secondary risk reduction strategy in patients with serious mental illness	Adults (308)	Motivational interviewing and skills building	Usual care	Risk taking behavior, HIV counseling and testing	Estimated completion, October 2014
Bull, 2008[171]* (Youthnet) United States	To develop and evaluate the effectiveness of tailored Web-based messages in promoting condom use	Young adults ages 18–25 y (1870)	Flash clips promoting condom use	General reproductive health information	Condom use	Completed December 2008
Colfax, 2011[172] United States	To determine the efficacy of a personalized cognitive risk reduction counseling intervention among episodic substance using men who have sex with men	Adult men who have sex with men (326)	Adapted, personalized cognitive risk reduction counseling	Standard HIV testing and information only	Unprotected sex acts, number of partners, STI incidence	Estimated completion, September 2012
Crosby, 2012[173] United States	To evaluate the efficacy of a brief, clinic-based, theory-guided intervention designed to reduce STI incidence and risk for HIV among young black men who have sex with men	Young males ages 15–29 y who have sex with males (620)	Weekly text messages, education program, and provision of condoms	Standard of care counseling plus provision of condoms	Unprotected sex acts	Estimated completion date, May 2016
DiClemente, 2012[174]* (Afiya) United States	To reduce risk for STI/HIV in young African American females	Adolescent African American females ages 14–20 y (701)	Group-based sexual health education program plus periodic telephone contacts designed to reinforce sexual health promotion	Group-based sexual health education program plus periodic telephone contacts to promote healthy dietary practices	STI incidence; condom use	Estimated completion, February 2013
Du Bois, 2012[175] (Keep It Up!) United States	To examine the efficacy of a Web-based HIV prevention intervention in reducing HIV risk behavior	Adult bisexual or gay men ages 18–24 y (660)	Web-based HIV prevention intervention	HIV/AIDS information only	TBD	NR
Fernandez, 2010[176] (Proyecto SOL) United States	To determine the efficacy of an HIV prevention behavioral intervention to reduce behaviors among Hispanic men who have sex with men	Adult Hispanic men who have sex with men (220)	Group-based intervention	HIV counseling and testing only	Unprotected sex acts	Completed March 2010

Appendix D. Ongoing or Recently Completed Studies

Study Country	Aim	Population (n)	Intervention Description	Control Description	Relevant Outcomes	Status
Garofalo, 2012[177] (LifeSkills) United States	To test the efficacy of a uniquely targeting HIV risk reduction intervention for young transgender women	Females ages 16–24 y (375)	Group-based manualized HIV prevention curriculum, HIV/STI testing and counseling	1) Group-based, manualized health promotion 2) Standard care	Unprotected sex acts	Estimated completion, December 2015
Gold, 2011[178]* (S.A.F.E.) United States	To assess the efficacy of a computer-assisted motivational intervention in reducing sexual risk-taking behaviors	Females ages 13–21 y (660)	One-on-one counseling guided by computer-generated personalized feedback	Didactic education counseling	Sexual and contraceptive behaviors	Completed December 2007
Houck, 2012[179] United States	To evaluate interventions for early adolescents with mental health issues to reduce risk behavior among	Adolescents ages 12–14 y (432)	Group intervention including affect management training and sexual health skills training	Group intervention including health information on a variety of relevant health topics	Sexual activity, condom use	Estimated completion, May 2014
Ickovics, 2012[180] United States	To determine the effectiveness of 2 prenatal care programs in reducing risk for HIV, STIs, and adverse perinatal outcomes in young women	Young adult females (1047)	CenteringPregnancy® plus group prenatal care with an HIV/STI prevention skill building component	1) CenteringPregnancy® group prenatal care 2) Usual prenatal care	STI incidence; sexual risk behavior	Estimated completion, December 2013
Kapungu, 2012[181] (Project STYLE) United States	To examine effectiveness of a family-based HIV prevention intervention targeting adolescents in psychiatric care	Adolescent psychiatric patients ages 13–18 y (305)	1) Family-based HIV prevention intervention 2) Adolescent-only HIV prevention intervention	Adolescent-only general health promotion	STI incidence, sexual behavior, drug/alcohol use	Completed, primary results not yet published
Lauby, 2011[182] (RISE) United States	To evaluate and determine the efficacy of an intervention to reduce acquiring or transmitting HIV among black bisexual men	Adult bisexual black men (250)	6 counseling sessions with trained counselor addressing stress, coping, and sexual health	1 standard HIV counseling session	Condom use	Estimated completion date NR; currently recruiting participants
Llewellyn, 2012[183] (PEPSE) United Kingdom	To examine the impact of motivational interviewing augmented with information provision and behavioral skills on risky sexual behaviors	Men who have sex with men (250)	Motivational interviewing augmented with information provision and behavioral skills	Usual care	Risky sexual practices, STI incidence	NR
Lescano, 2012[184] United States	To determine the efficacy of a Latino family-based HIV prevention intervention	Parent and adolescent dyads (640)	1 HIV-specific, family-based workshop with a followup booster session	1 family-based general health promotion workshop with a followup booster session	Sexual activity status, unprotected sex acts, condom use	Estimated completion, December 2014
Miller, 2009[185] (SOLVE-IT study) United States	To evaluate the effectiveness of an interactive virtual environment computer game in reducing risky sexual behaviors in men who have sex with men	Men who have sex with men (4000)	Interactive virtual computer game (decisionmaking, skill building)	Waitlist	Unprotected sex	Estimated completion, December 2012
Morokoff, 2008[186]* United States	To evaluate a new program designed to increase condom use	Adults ages 18–44 y (534)	Computer-delivered individual feedback and tailored manual	General HIV information	Condom use, unprotected sex acts	Completed October 2007
Murphy, 2011[187] United States	To determine the preliminary efficacy of a family-based HIV prevention intervention in adolescent girls	Adolescent girls ages 15–19 y (168)	Family-based HIV risk reduction prevention intervention	No intervention	Unprotected sex acts	Completed December 2006

Appendix D. Ongoing or Recently Completed Studies

Study Country	Aim	Population (n)	Intervention Description	Control Description	Relevant Outcomes	Status
Noar, 2011[188,189] (TIPSS) United States	To test a computerized HIV/STI prevention program among heterosexual African Americans	Adults ages 18–29 y (312)	Computerized intervention program based on the Attitude-Social-Influence efficacy model, tailored feedback and interactive activities for skill building (guided by social cognitive theory)	Wait-list control	Condom use	Completed February 2012
O'Donnell, 2010[190] United States	To evaluate a brief, video-based, group intervention designed to reduce sexual risk-taking among Latino men who have sex with men	Men ages 18–49 y who have sex with men (370)	Video on HIV prevention education	HIV counseling and testing	Sexual risk behavior	Completed, November 2009
Patterson, 2012[191*] United States	To evaluate the effectiveness of a sexual risk reduction intervention in reducing sexual risk behavior in methamphetamine users	Adult drug users (400)	Trifocal cognitive behavioral therapy and social skills training counseling	Standard care	Unprotected sex, STI incidence, HIV serostatus	Completed August 2012
Rizzo, 2011[192] (Date SMART) United States	To develop and test a group-based preventive intervention to reduce dating violence and sexual risk behavior among adolescent females	Adolescent females (100)	Cognitive behavioral intervention (Skills to Manager Aggression in Relationships for Teens) for dating violence and HIV prevention	Psychoeducational dating violence and HIV prevention	Unprotected sexual activity	Estimated completion, February 2014
Shegog, 2011[193] (It's Your Game... Keep It Real) United States	To delay sexual activity among American Indian/Alaskan Native youth	Adolescents ages 12–14 y (1200)	Culturally-adapted, Web-based HIV, STI, and pregnancy prevention curriculum	Web-based science education program	Delay onset of sexual activity; other changes in sexual behaviors (e.g., reduce number of partners)	Estimated completion, June 2014
Sperling, 2005[194*] United States	To evaluate the efficacy of the MISTERS intervention for men post-release from jail	Men ages 18–60 y (300)	Cognitive behavioral skill building multisession intervention	Control	Change in risk behaviors, STI incidence	Completed, June 2004
Sullivan, 2010[195] (Project RED) United States	To evaluate the impact of enhanced sexual risk reduction counseling	Adult opioid users ages 18–65 y (114)	Enhanced sexual risk reduction, individual, gender-specific counseling, including skill building	Standard physician counseling	Condom use, unprotected sex acts, number of sex partners, STI incidence	Completed, June 2011
University of Pittsburgh, 2012[196] (StARSS) United States	To determine the efficacy of a text-message program to reduce risky sexual behavior in young females identified from the emergency department	Women ages 18–25 y (68)	Weekly lifestyle counseling text messages assessing risky sexual encounters and providing feedback	Usual care	Unprotected sex, condom use	Completed July 2012
Wechsberg, 2012[197] (Young Women's CoOp Study) United States	To evaluate the efficacy of a cultural-, age-, and gender-focused HIV prevention intervention in reducing risk behaviors	Young adult African American females ages 16–19 y (237)	Individual and group counseling sessions	Attention control (nutrition intervention)	Condom use	Completed August 2012

Appendix D. Ongoing or Recently Completed Studies

Study Country	Aim	Population (n)	Intervention Description	Control Description	Relevant Outcomes	Status
Wu, 2012[198] (Connect 'n Unite) United States	To test whether participants in a couple-based behavioral prevention intervention engage in lower risk HIV/STI behaviors	Adult black male drug users who have sex with men (480)	Couples-based behavioral HIV/STI prevention	Couples-based wellness promotion	STI incidence, sexual HIV risk behavior	Estimated completion, February 2015
Zule, 2011[199] (CATCH) United States	To pilot test a cue card driven, computer-assisted, risk reduction intervention on sexual risk behaviors	Adult men who have sex with men (120)	Education and skill building tailored to each participant's demographics, risk behaviors, and biological test results	Waitlist	Unprotected sex acts	Completed July 2012

*Study was also identified as ongoing in the previous review.

www.ingramcontent.com/pod-product-compliance
Lightning Source LLC
Chambersburg PA
CBHW081726170526
45167CB00009B/3713